200

REBUILDING SERGEANT PECK

HOW I PUT BODY AND SOUL BACK TOGETHER AFTER AFGHANISTAN

JOHN M. PECK,

Dava Guerin, *and* Terry Bivens

Forewords by Gary Sinise and Jennifer Griffin

Skyhorse Publishing

To my fallen Marines—you are the true heroes. And to my donor and his family, who, after his passing, gave me his arms and a chance to pursue my dreams.

Skyhorse Publishing books may be purchased in bulk at special discounts for sales promotion, corporate gifts, fund-raising, or educational purposes. Special editions can also be created to specifications. For details, contact the Special Sales Department, Skyhorse Publishing, 307 West 36th Street, 11th Floor, New York, NY 10018 or info@skyhorsepublishing.com.

Skyhorse® and Skyhorse Publishing® are registered trademarks of Skyhorse Publishing, Inc.®, a Delaware corporation.

Visit our website at www.skyhorsepublishing.com.

10 9 8 7 6 5 4 3 2 1

Library of Congress Cataloging-in-Publication Data is available on file.

Cover design by Qualcom
Cover photo courtesy of Jessica Peck

ISBN: 978-1-5107-4065-5
Ebook ISBN: 978-1-5107-4066-2

Printed in the United States of America

TABLE OF CONTENTS

Foreword

Gary Sinise, actor, humanitarian, and founder of the Gary Sinise Foundation

I MET SGT. JOHN PECK IN THE FALL OF 2010; HE HAS BEEN AN INSPIRATION TO me ever since. John has rebuilt his body and soul, and his is a compelling story of determination, persistence, and service.

After committing to build homes for the first two surviving quadruple amputees from the War on Terror, Brendan Marrocco and Todd Nicely, we received a third and most distressing call. On May 24, 2010, Sgt. John Peck had finished sweeping a compound with a metal detector checking for bombs, when he stepped on an IED. He became America's third surviving quadruple amputee.

As I had pledged my support for Brendan and Todd by building smart homes for them, I wanted to meet John to see how I could help him and learn more about his injuries and needs going forward. That was the summer of 2010. While his mother was staying with him at Walter Reed, still John was struggling physically and mentally. He was battling depression, and it was important for me to let him know that he was not alone and was supported. Despite the severity of his injuries, it was obvious to me that John was special. You could see the determination in his eyes, and I knew—though his recovery would be long and painful—he would tackle it like the consummate Marine he is.

So, I invited John and his mom to attend our 2011 Salute to the Troops event in Vegas. Fortunately, they were able to get away from the hospital, and I was happy to see John smile and have some welcome relief from his pain. We offered to raise funds to help build a smart home for him as well, and this was very early on in the creation of my foundation. It was no simple matter to raise the funds necessary for each smart home project. But our heroes deserve this and more, and I wanted to do everything I could to help. One of the ways we did this was by performing fund-raising concerts. We did one each for Brendan and Todd within a year of their injuries. They both attended their tribute concerts, and they were great celebrations of their service to our country. Through these efforts, we were able to raise a portion of the money to begin their building projects, as well as raise awareness for what we were doing. John would be our next endeavor, and I couldn't be happier.

In the beginning, John wasn't sure whether he wanted to live in his home state of Illinois, so, his concert wasn't able to materialize as quickly as the others. In the summer of 2011, the father of a fallen soldier, Hector Castro, reached out to me. His son, U.S. Army Specialist A.J. Castro, had been killed while fighting in Afghanistan. Hector wanted to do something to honor his fallen son. So, I suggested we raise some funds and put them into home building projects for our wounded. Hector liked the idea, and we set up a tribute concert in A.J.'s name at a small club in Agoura Hills, California, which raised $75,000. With Hector's blessing, we put the proceeds toward John's house, along with a plaque that we eventually placed in John's new home in honor of A.J. In 2012, we raised even more money for John at the annual *Rockin' For the Troops* concert that I host and perform with my Lt. Dan Band each year in Wheaton, Illinois, in support of *Operation Support Our Troops America*. As John was originally from Illinois, I asked the organization to donate $125,000 raised at that concert to go toward John's home. Finally, we raised an additional $100,000 for John from my pal Clint Eastwood, who quietly wanted to support my efforts on behalf of our wounded.

November 11, 2012, Veterans Day, was a wonderful day. We handed over the keys to John for his new home built in Fredericksburg, Virginia. I was unable to attend the ceremony myself, but in video and photographs, I saw so many smiles from John that day. Smiles that were absent just a few years before. And that was beautiful to see.

Getting to know John over the years and watching him go from such a low point in the beginning to such resilience and strength has been remarkable. I have seen him at many of my concerts including Ft. Belvoir, and a concert to raise funds in Pennsylvania for Adam Keys, one of John's friends. Only a few months before, we handed over keys to John for his home.

I have continued to stay in touch with him over the years and marvel at his courage. John has not only rebuilt his life, but now with his new arms, his dreams of being a professional chef seem unstoppable. Most of all, John knows the meaning of service firsthand. Not just his military service, but helping those in need. That's why I believe John's book, *Rebuilding Sergeant Peck: How I Put Body and Soul Back Together after Afghanistan,* will inspire anyone regardless of whether they serve in the military or not. I'm proud to call John my pal. John has spent his life giving back in so many ways, and for that reason, he is my hero.

—*Gary Sinise*

FOREWORD

Jennifer Griffin, Fox News national security correspondent

REMEMBER MEETING SGT. JOHN PECK FOR THE FIRST TIME IN 2012. HE WAS in the audience at the Lt. Dan Band concert in Beaufort, South Carolina, where Gary Sinise and his band were playing for an audience of wounded veterans and their caregivers. They had been brought together by the Independence Fund. John is one of only a handful of quadruple amputees from the wars in Iraq and Afghanistan. He has an irrepressible boyish outlook. We all danced together under the stars, as Gary and his band played. What John didn't realize was that his youthful wish for a better wheelchair that wouldn't get stuck in the mud launched a movement that night. Now, nearly 1,500 veterans and their families' lives have been changed forever because of his desire to get back outside on his wooded lot in rural Virginia. It is one of the most beautiful grassroots initiatives that this patriotic country has ever produced.

John told the organizers that night that he had his eye on a wheelchair with tank-like treads that he could use on his land. These "Trackchairs" cost a princely sum: about $15,000. There were many hands that night in taking this "wish" and turning it into a reality. Perhaps it was Captain John "Woody" Woodall, a veteran firefighter who was dressed as Elvis and sang the Star-Spangled Banner that night, who fanned the spark. Or Kyle Johnson, the owner of a medical device company who placed the first bid that made the Trackchair a reality. Steve Danyluk, the former Marine American Airlines pilot, deserves credit for taking this idea and running with it.

Months later at the Walter Reed Christmas party, the first Trackchairs were ready to be delivered. Kyle Johnson flew up from Beaufort. Woody was dressed as Elvis, and John Peck was in the Warrior Café at Walter Reed with the other veterans and their families. Some were missing limbs. Others were suffering from traumatic brain injuries. My daughters, Annalise and Amelia, accompanied me and were handing out wrapped presents to some of the warriors and the children of those warriors who were living at Walter Reed in Bethesda while their parents were being treated. Some had been there for months, even years. When it was time to present John Peck his Trackchair, Kyle Johnson stepped up again.

Seeing the look on the face of John, who was doing wheelies with his chair in front of the hospital as though it were his first BMX bike, or the looks on the faces of those amputees who wanted a chair but stared at them longingly as though they were a red Lamborghini, Kyle donated money for another Trackchair to be given away at the Christmas party. My daughters were sitting at a table with a double amputee named Kevin. They had offered him a space at their table when he was wheeling toward them with a plate full of food. Woody asked them who should get the next Trackchair. They shouted in unison: Kevin. That was the beginning of what has become a movement championed by Bill O'Reilly, the former Fox anchor. But John Peck introduced everyone to these Trackchairs.

A few weeks later, I went down to Fredericksburg, Virginia, to his Smart Home built by the Gary Sinise Foundation, to see John use his Trackchair. Before our cameras began rolling, he wanted to have a cigarette. I looked at him and, a cancer survivor myself, said, "You know they can kill you." He was nonplussed. John then proceeded to hook his Trackchair up to his SUV and pull it up the driveway. He whooped and hollered as he went rolling over the hills in his front yard. The sheer joy on his face, the sheer will to live and live well, is what makes John such an inspiration. He showed me videos of him skydiving after losing his limbs. He went scuba diving. He cooks. He dated on Match.com. He came to speak at my daughters' school and enthralled their sixth- and seventh-grade classes. He told them how he wants to have a double arm transplant. The children of John Eaton School in Washington, D.C., then held a car wash and raised $1,100.01 for the surgery. You could hear a pin drop when he spoke to the students. None of them have forgotten that visit. He described being blown up in Helmand Province on May 24, 2010: "All I could feel was this immense amount of pain and burning. I came back to, and I could feel the rotor wash from the helicopter." He said to himself, "I don't want to die here. I can't die here. This is Afghanistan. This place sucks." He woke up two-and-a-half months later in Bethesda Naval Hospital. He found out he was pronounced dead once and had more than twenty-eight surgeries.

Marine Sgt. John Peck is a survivor, but he is also a thriver. His story still makes me smile. I am so grateful that he entered our lives.

INTRODUCTION

S ERGEANT PECK REPORTING FOR DUTY, SIR. YEP, THAT'S ME, BUT THIS TIME I wasn't serving in the United States Marine Corps, but sitting around with my wife and some friends cooking pizzas. My job was to throw on the pepperoni and mushrooms. I can't chop up the onions or shred the cheese the way I would like. But I'm doing damn good for someone who's using what more than two years ago were someone else's arms and hands. And I'm certain that one day I'll slice, dice, and shred with the best of them.

You may have seen me on television or read about me in the newspaper or on social media. I'm the Marine sergeant who lost both arms and legs in the War on Terror, one of only five other quadruple amputees serving in the military. I'm also one of the roughly eighty people worldwide to receive a successful double arm transplant and one of the fewer still having an above-the-elbow attachment. I did that in the fall of 2016, thanks to the great doctors at Brigham and Women's Hospital in Boston. Before this ground-breaking surgery, I could not hold my wife's hand. Now I can.

Being a quadruple amputee isn't fun. It's hell, that's for sure. But now that I have my new arms, things are getting better. Little by little, I can move them the way I want and do simple things that I couldn't before, like combing my hair or washing myself in the shower. And there isn't a day that goes by that I don't look down at what I call *our* arms and think about my donor and what he did for me. His family's sacrifice is something I will never forget.

I know that as time goes by, I'll be able to do a lot more; I plan to cook dinner for all my family and friends someday.

Life, I guess you could say, has thrown a lot at me. My dad abandoned me even before I was born. Growing up wasn't easy, but is it for anyone? After high school, I found a home in the United States Marine Corps, but my challenges were only beginning. In 2007, on my first tour in Iraq, my buddies and I were returning from a grueling day-long patrol when we rounded a corner in a seven-ton armored truck and rolled over an IED. I was manning the M240 machine gun. The blast smashed my head into the gun.

As a result, I suffered a traumatic brain injury (TBI), as well as vision, balance, and hearing problems. My memory was shot. When my first wife came to visit me in the hospital, I had no idea who she was, much less that I had married her. Or why I had married her. I tried everything I could to rekindle my feelings for her, or even develop new ones. But nothing seemed to work, and eventually, we got divorced.

But as I said, I'm a Marine. I love the job. I signed up to fight, and, TBI and all, I convinced the Marine Corps to send me back into battle. This time it was Afghanistan. And this time it was even worse.

It was May 24, 2010. I was walking a patrol in the infamous Helmand Province. I was clearing a compound with a metal detector and remember my sergeant asking me if I found anything yet. I told him I didn't. I took one more step and yelled to my sergeant, "I found one!" The other guys in my unit started running, and my sergeant ran toward me to pull me away. He never made it. The next step I took changed everything. The IED blew off both of my legs and part of my right arm. Apparently, my sergeant told my mom later that it was chaos. Luckily, all my sergeant suffered was some hearing loss. I didn't make out so well.

It's hard to remember everything that's happened in the years since. Hell, it's sometimes hard for me to remember anything at all, thanks to my traumatic brain injury. But I'm told it involved some twenty-eight surgeries, a bout with a flesh-eating fungus, and a collapsed stent that eventually claimed the only limb I had left, my left arm. My blood pressure dropped to dangerous levels during some of those surgeries. A few times, I almost died. And that's just a taste of what I've been through.

But I'm alive, very much alive. I have two new arms, thanks to a man whose death I mourn every day. Though I can't reveal his name because of the donor's family wishes, his father told me that he was a caring and talented young man. He was only in his twenties when he died of a rare brain disease, and thanks to his generosity, I was fortunate to receive his beautiful arms. He will always be a part of me as long as I live. I also have a beautiful and caring wife, Jessica, who loves me. I have a mission in life—to become a great chef, motivational speaker, and a help to other wounded warriors just like me. And I have this book.

So why am I writing it? Well, it's not for the publicity or a chance to be famous. Anyone who knows me realizes that I hate the spotlight. When I'm thrust into it, I kind of shut down, lower my head, and hope it ends soon. Sure, I did some publicity with the hospital in Boston when I had my arm transplant, but I did that to let people in similar situations know there was a way to actually get your arms back; I'm living proof. And to encourage every American citizen to become an organ donor.

I didn't do it for the money, either. No, I'm writing this book to give hope to all those people who run into something terrible in their lives and can't see their way past it. God knows I've had many times when I could have just quit, just said, "Screw it." But I pushed on like any Marine or soldier would. No pain, no gain.

I hope through this book readers can learn from my unusual and challenging life experiences. My story will take them from my chaotic childhood and troubled adolescence to my search for purpose, a purpose I found in the United States Marine Corps. But after all the pride and accomplishment I gained in the Corps, my life suddenly fell to depths no one should experience—losing all my limbs and searching for a way to kill myself. Through it all, however, I've emerged as a stronger and more empathetic human being—truly rebuilt, including my new arms. I want readers to know that things will always get better, to have faith, and to try to have a sense of humor about it all. If I can achieve my goals with all that I've been through, anyone can.

Now as I said, I'm a Marine. Don't expect me to write flowery phrases or to lay some heavy positive thinking rap on you like some leatherneck Norman Vincent Peale. People overcome terrible adversity for many different reasons. Mine was a rock-hard, almost genetically engineered will to survive, a drive that has pushed me to overcome everything I faced. It wavered only once, that time at Walter Reed when I was suicidal. I even came up with a plan to take my wheelchair to the top floor of the building where I was living and let it tumble down the steps. I wanted to end my pain.

Then, the day before I was going to call it quits, I looked out the window and saw a soldier with no legs—just like me—sitting in his wheelchair. I remember imagining he was on his way to wheel that chair right into the busy traffic outside the base. But then I saw who I assumed was his wife and a little child walking over to meet him. She put the child on his lap, and they left, her pushing the chair and all of them smiling and laughing. I thought, *Hell, if he can have a wife and child and be happy, so could I.*

My core, my fiery will to survive, had kicked back in. If I can find that will, you can, too.

Before I start, though, let me say one quick, but important, thing. The traumatic brain injury (TBI) I mentioned earlier affects me deeply to this day. TBI affects different people in different ways, but for me, it made remembering parts of my life painful, challenging, and, in some cases, almost impossible. It's like a clock with a few gear teeth missing; sometimes there are jolting, maddening gaps. I've tried to fill those gaps with some help from others and with the insights I've gained by surviving my tumultuous life and emerging a stronger, more tolerant, and better person.

PREFACE

Rebuilt: Announcing My New Arms

THE BIG DAY IS FINALLY HERE. TODAY, I'LL MEET THE PRESS FOR THE FIRST time following my double arm transplant. I hate this kind of stuff. But the office of strategic communications at Brigham and Women's Hospital in Boston, Massachusetts, stressed the importance of telling my story for the first time to the world. I can't stand being the center of attention, but this time is different. I'm speaking for two people now, not just one.

It took a little while before I was ready for this moment. My doctors had to wait to make sure my new arms weren't rejected and that I didn't have any signs of infection. Plus, the pain sucked, and there was no way right after my surgery that I could speak in public without babbling my brains out, thanks to all the pain meds and just the normal stages of recovery from such a major surgery.

My mom told me about this type of surgery soon after my injury. Thank goodness she did. I did my own research, as well. My girlfriend, now my wife, Jessica, was there by my side all the way. Though at the time she only knew me for six months, she was my rock. She helped me get ready to travel to the hospital in Boston from my home in Virginia, helped me understand what was involved in such a groundbreaking surgery, and, most of all, was my support system. I couldn't have done this without her. Jess used to call me her "penguin." Now don't get the wrong idea. What she meant was that emperor penguins meet their soul mates and stay together for life; Jess and I have no intention of messing with Mother Nature.

The morning of the press conference, which was held in a large room at Brigham, I felt a million different emotions. Just a few months before, I was a quadruple amputee. While it wasn't a cakewalk living without arms and legs, plus suffering from a traumatic brain injury, I could still grab a plate from the cabinet thanks to my prosthetic arms and only needed help with things like putting on my shorts, showering, or running errands. I also needed someone there to help me with some other tasks that go along with being basically semi-independent. There were some days that I felt like shit. It was humiliating having to ask someone to help me with the most basic things like brushing my teeth, washing my hair, and putting on my shorts. What a sucker punch for a guy who was a strong, tough Marine and now has to be treated like a helpless baby.

So, there I was ready to announce to the world what previously I thought was only a pipe dream.

Before we entered the room for the press conference, I was so keyed up that I said every swear word I could think of, just to get the tension out of my system. "Fuck, fuck, fuck, shit, shit, shit," I repeated over and over. "Goddamnit, motherfucker, shit, shit, shit," I continued to mumble to myself. I'm sure anyone who heard me cursing like that thought I was nuts! Jess, the doctors, and the chief communications officer heard me.

What they were worried about was me—a Marine after all—having an open microphone and saying something off-color out of pure nervousness. They said something like this: "Hey John, we're going to wire you up right now, so as soon as you enter the room, watch what you say, or they'll hear you."

Fortunately, the Brigham communications team prepared me for interviews, and that did help to get me ready for this moment. I insisted, however, that I write my own remarks. They also prepped me for the fact that there would be plenty of media there and gave me some questions they assumed the press was bound to ask. We practiced my speech over and over in a kind of mock-interview setting, and someone remarked that I needed to read it with more feeling. I get it. It had to be done. But this was my body. My new arms. My story. And there was no way that I was going to convey someone else's version of how I felt at this critical moment. It was as if I were having an out-of-body experience. Here I was going to tell the world my story, but now with someone else's arms attached to my stubs. I felt my donor's presence as I tried to hold back my tears.

As the press conference was ready to begin, I glanced over at all the reporters in the room. It was surreal. As my doctors and I sat behind a rectangular table that had microphones for us to answer the reporters' questions, I was scared. But it was weird that I wasn't scared for me, but more like overwhelmed that this moment was finally here. While I was basically happy, it hit me hard that someone had to die to give me this gift. I vowed I never was going to waste it.

While I did have my talking points ready to roll, I made a split-second decision to go for it and just tell these people what was in my heart. I said something like this: "Following my surgery, I looked down at my arms, and the minute I saw them, I knew they were a perfect match. The skin color was perfect. It seemed natural, and they were just like mine. The detail of my fingers was perfect, too." I also told them that I was excited to be able to wear the bracelet on my new wrist that has the name of Cpl. Larry D. Harris, my fallen brother, on it. Let me tell you about him. Cpl. Harris died on July 1. He was a squad leader, like me, and was pinned down by machine gun fire. One of his men received small arms fire and was wounded. Cpl. Harris, without concern for his own life, rushed toward his men and immediately applied first aid. After it was decided to move his men to the CASEVAC site, Cpl. Larry Harris stepped on a pressure plate IED. His body absorbed most of the blast. He was awarded the Silver Star posthumously. We have a code in the Marines that says that we don't look at skin color, race, or ethnicity. You are my brother as long as you would take a bullet for me.

I wear Cpl. Harris's bracelet, not just because he was killed in battle, but to celebrate his life and all the other guys who lost their lives, as well. I will always love my buddies and never forget them. And now that I have my arms, *our* arms, I explained to the media, that bracelet will be the first thing that I put on when I'm able.

I felt the tears welling up inside me as I looked down at *our* arms with the world watching. My donor was a young man who died of a rare and fatal brain disease, though during the press conference, I didn't know that. In fact, I knew nothing about my donor at all. His parents only came forward after they saw me at the press conference and heard me talking about their son. Soon after that, my donor's father sent me a long and heartfelt message on my Facebook page. It simply said: "Hey, John, I have to tell you a story; we have a lot in common." It was mind-blowing.

I realized my donor gave me a gift that he should have never have had to give. Because of his passing—and his courageous decision to donate his eyes, heart, kidney, liver, and skin, plus his two arms—I was able to become almost whole again. I made a promise to his parents that day at the press conference. I said: "I won't let you down. I will do right by your son and fulfill my dreams of becoming a chef, thanks to his sacrifice." While it was too painful for my donor's parents to attend the press conference, I know they heard my words; I meant every one of them.

I'm no hero. But this guy, my brother, my organ donor, is mine. Together, we will overcome the tragedies in our lives. We will rebuild each other, one touch at a time.

ONE

JUST THE TWO OF US

I CAN'T REALLY TELL MY STORY PROPERLY WITHOUT FIRST A FEW WORDS ABOUT my mom, Norma. Because for much of my life, it was the two of us against the world. So, bear with me. It's definitely worth it.

She loves our country, loves the flag, and has stuck with me no matter what. I guess you could say that our relationship is like many others between parents and their kids, sometimes great, often challenging. The funny thing is that we're very much alike. We're both stubborn, smart, energetic, opinionated, and don't take any shit from anyone. We both had a rough time growing up. There was emotional and physical abuse. Financial problems. Homelessness. Abandonment.

But despite those hardships, my mom and I were always superpatriotic and caring people. We both love the military and would do anything to lend a hand to someone down on their luck. I think my mom and my Uncle Toby had an influence because of their service and what I saw growing up, but I'm the kind of guy who is just a natural protector. I care about people and have a strong sense of duty. While my mom coped with stress more seriously, I did it with humor, so maybe that's where we differ. But no matter what we had to deal with, we are survivors. It seems to be in our DNA.

My mom never had the money to go to college. But she was smart enough to get into any school if she could have afforded the tuition. She once told me a story about when she was a kid and how much she loved our country, and when she was in the fifth grade, she dreamed about singing the

1

Star-Spangled Banner. I guess you could say that like so many Americans who love this country, having an opportunity to serve was its own kind of patriotism. My mom was a proud American.

Her military career began a year before I was born. Since my mom loved the medical field, she visited a Marine recruiter, hoping to be able to use that passion in the Marine Corps. The recruiter quickly shot her down. "Ma'am, we don't let ladies do any medical work," he told her. She was shocked but wouldn't give up. The guy did give her some advice, though, suggesting the Navy or the National Guard. But the Army got her first when she learned about a program that offered medical training. She signed up on the spot. My mom's tenaciousness and resolve are probably the qualities I most inherited from her. And boy, would they come in handy as I had to overcome more than my share of obstacles.

My mom was slated to be stationed at Ft. Polk, Louisiana, but in June 1984 she got in a terrible motorcycle accident and couldn't make her departure date. After she healed up, she went back to Chicago to the recruiter's office and filled out the paperwork to give it another try. They issued her a new departure date, but she told the recruiter that if they didn't have a medical position available, she wasn't going. "You better find me what I want in the medical field, or that's it," she told him. Sure enough, he found her the perfect job—a combat medical specialist. She was now officially in the U.S. Army.

My mom was never deployed overseas like me. When she was eighteen, she met my dad (though I don't think he deserves that title) and became pregnant with me. They met in Texas when he was in the Marines. She fell hard for him, as she told me once, but they were essentially teenagers, so I'm sure there wasn't much more than chemistry between them. His name was Mike. What an asshole. When my mom told him about the pregnancy, he denied it was his baby and backed out of taking responsibility and marrying my mom. He said some nonsense like, "It's your baby; I'm nothing but the sperm donor."

So, she was a single mom for all my childhood and adolescence. I never met Mike until I was nine years old, and that was a disaster. I'll tell you more about him later, but for now, suffice to say it may have been better for me, in the long run, to have him remain anonymous.

After the Army learned she was pregnant, they transferred her to Louisiana, where she worked in a pediatric unit of a local hospital. There she met a guy named John. They had a whirlwind romance and got married, even though she was pregnant with me. They decided to move to Florida to be closer to his family. Then, on September 13, 1985, I was born.

My mom always wanted me to be the kind of person that helps other people, not just someone who looks out for himself. For as long as I can remember, my mom and I would stop the car to help someone who needed medical attention if there wasn't an ambulance on the scene. I'm sure that was one of the reasons that I've always been drawn to doing acts of kindness and helping others in need.

My mom reminded me recently that we did that sort of thing from the time I was a young child to when I was a teenager; literally, hundreds of times, if not more. My mom always believed that it was her responsibility to help other people and break the cycle of abuse that she suffered during her own childhood.

In fact, she was doing it even before I was born. She and John were driving home from work when she noticed a car on the side of the road with two feet sticking out of the back window. My mom immediately knew what was happening. The "feet" meant someone was about to give birth. They pulled over in a nanosecond, and my mom jumped out of the car and got into her Army medical mode. Remember, my mom was seven months pregnant at the time. In just about an hour or so, she helped a complete stranger deliver a healthy baby.

My mom told me that the new mother said to her after the baby was born, "I can't believe you're not sitting here next to me delivering your own baby."

Of course, I don't remember much from that time, but my mom told me that when I was about one, she came home only to find that John had packed up his stuff and moved out.

That still baffles me to this day how someone who was obviously such a caring and kind person could be totally abandoned, without warning, and left to fend for herself. He was a bolter, a real shithead!

Clearly, my mom had no luck with men. I think this was because of her own issues she experienced growing up. When you have two highly dysfunctional parents, and you add to that alcohol and verbal and physical abuse, how the hell could my mom trust anyone again? And, while I was too young to know it, I had only gotten my first taste of the tumult that would follow.

So, there we were, just the two of us.

Times were tough. My mom always had trouble paying the bills. She had to work two jobs just to put food on the table, while at the same time serving as a field medic in the Army Reserves. Even though I was still in diapers, I believe I somehow absorbed the tension swirling around me. Early experiences, they say, can affect a person throughout their life. From what I was told, I cried for my mom when she had to do her one weekend a month Reserve duty, driving up to Wisconsin and leaving me behind.

In the reserves, her duties were to keep all the equipment clean and stocked and to make sure the unit's four ambulances were ready for action. But after about four years or so, she decided to quit. The captain of her unit promised her when she signed up that she would be sent to nursing school. When she asked him when she was going to start, he told her: "Ma'am, we're not doing that anymore." She was royally pissed. On Monday morning, my mom called the recruiter and said: "I want out." Like me, when my mom makes up her mind, that's it.

To make ends meet after leaving the reserves, she did a lot of nursing jobs—home care and whatnot. She also worked for a temporary agency, a medical office, was a babysitter, and even did some modeling. She told me stories about those times, and how some of her trickiest situations included finding a competent and trustworthy babysitter for me.

When we moved from Florida back to Rockford, Illinois, we lived in an old farmhouse with my grandparents. My mom had an off-and-on relationship with my grandmother; they fought a lot. Years later, my mom told me about the abuse she suffered at the hands of both my grandparents. My grandfather was an alcoholic, and my grandmother was verbally abusive to my mom, and even occasionally physically abusive. My mom told me that my grandmother once got so mad at her that she made her stick her head in the oven. Thank God it wasn't turned on.

My babysitters always seemed to be an issue between my mom and grandmother. My mom often worked two jobs, so a babysitter was a necessity. After several tries, my mom finally found a sitter she trusted. But even that went bad. One time, around Valentine's Day, I had a fever. My mom had to miss work for a couple of days but finally decided that my fever had broken and it was okay for her to leave me with the babysitter. She told the babysitter that if I ran a fever above one hundred and one, to call her immediately. My mom gave the sitter her number at work, with explicit instructions for what to do if my fever returned.

Since it was a few days before Valentine's Day, the guy she was dating at the time wanted to take her out to dinner. She told him that she could only go if I was not still sick. She even gave the babysitter the number of the restaurant so she could call her in case I got worse. My mom said she felt okay with everything and headed out for dinner with her date. At around seven that night, the babysitter called my mom and told her that my temperature had spiked to one hundred and three degrees. She also informed her that she called my grandmother and that they were taking me to the emergency room at the hospital where my mom worked. My mom was furious. I ended up fine, but the incident only led to more fighting between my mom and my grandmother. Needless to say, I never saw the babysitter again.

My grandmother threatened to take me away from my mom because of that incident, and that wasn't the last time that would happen. And what I didn't know at the time was that my mom was pregnant from her time with John with a baby girl, which she decided to give up for adoption. I often wonder what she is doing and what she has become in life. I guess some things not even a Marine like me can answer.

Despite my mom's difficulties with male relationships, she never gave up trying to find the right man and hoped to settle down once she finally found him. She started seeing this new guy, and, before long, she decided to marry him. I guess she believed it was the right thing to do—marrying and moving out of the farmhouse and in with this guy—but it ushered in one of the worst periods of my young life.

Her second husband, Adam, was a cop. I have trouble remembering how he looked, other than he was dark-haired and I think Hispanic. One thing I'm sure of: he had a real mean streak where I was concerned. I guess I was around four by then. I can't remember what I did, but I do remember Adam putting his hand over my nose and mouth so I couldn't breathe. What a sweetheart. This guy did stuff like that to me on a regular basis. Like the time he threw my dinner on the floor and made me eat it like a dog. Or when he made me sit alone on the cold basement floor when my mom was working cleaning offices in the evening. His constant verbal and physical abuse left me terrified and always on high alert. All I can recall from that time was that I feared for my life, never knowing what would trigger Adam's rages. I can't remember if I had nightmares or trouble eating or anything. But I do remember that I walked on eggshells around him and steered clear of him when I could.

Still, things continued to go from bad to worse. But I was afraid to tell my mom. I'm not exactly sure why I felt that way at the time, other than I was afraid of what Adam would do once I let the cat out of the bag. She never knew at the time what living hell I was going through. Looking back, and knowing how my mom always protected me, I wish I had spoken up sooner.

Adam's daughter was no picnic, either. Teenage girls can be cruel, and she could have been the lead character in the movie *Mean Girls*. She would tease me about everything and seemed to get enormous pleasure by taunting me, nonstop. Once it got so bad that I grabbed a knife, gently dragging it over her knee. I was only about five years old. I don't think I really intended to stab her, but a knife is serious business. Adam was furious. I'm surprised he didn't go wild on me. His ex-wife, meanwhile, even threatened to call the cops on me. But looking back, I realize that, even as a five-year-old, I did what I had to do to survive. I kept my mouth shut and took whatever Adam dished out. That may have been the first time my genetically instilled survival gene would kick in. As you'll see, that gene would serve me well in the times to come.

Life with Adam was so traumatizing for me that I was numb and paralyzed emotionally. I mean, who wouldn't be? I'm sure being treated like a dog, literally and figuratively, left its scars. But still, I never told my mom about the abuse Adam leveled on me. That is, until she and Adam split and we moved out. I believe she left because Adam was not what she had expected in a husband, and I'm sure on some subconscious level, she knew that he and I were not getting along at all. Now, as an adult, it is so apparent to me how abuse negatively affects a person. How can you be happy and secure when you are always looking over your shoulder for the next terrible thing to happen? My mom grew up that way, and it's hard to break those patterns unless you do some serious soul-searching.

Since we literally had no place to go, we moved into a women's shelter. When I got up the nerve to tell mom about Adam's abuse, she went berserk. She talked to the people in the shelter and asked them if she should call the police. They advised her against that since first, Adam would then know where we were, and second, he was a cop. The likelihood he would find out, and maybe retaliate, would be high. It wasn't worth the risk.

For me, it was good to finally get this off my chest, but I did feel guilty in a way that I was making my mom feel so bad. And Adam lingered in my mind, the thought of him back then making my stomach knot. Some twenty-eight years later, I think that I was more afraid of him than any person since, including those terrorists we were trained to kill in Iraq and Afghanistan.

Mom eventually divorced this bastard. But even though Adam was no longer around, his abuse left a deep scar. I felt him in my bones for years afterward. Adam did his best to bully me into a kid who feared his own shadow. But, there is something inside me—no matter what I've endured—that takes a deep breath and changes course, coming back even stronger than before. Mom was a little slower to bounce back. No matter what shitty thing happened to her, she always endured. It was my destiny to follow suit.

It took a while, but Mom eventually earned enough money to get us out of the shelter and into our own apartment. In fact, we went through a series of apartments. And while I don't remember much about any of them, I do remember her rules. There were lots of them. Like I had to be patriotic and respect the flag, do my chores, and not get in any trouble. My mom told me that she had to be "creative" with me, since I was a rambunctious kid. One of my punishments was having to do jumping jacks and sit-ups. If I was really bad, she would make me stand at attention in the corner of the room. When you're that young, that's serious punishment.

And, of course, money was always an issue. I still remember how my mom and I were incredibly careful with what money we had. Every Sunday morning, we would wake up, go to the store, and buy a few local newspapers. When we got back home, we would eat breakfast, then cut out all the food coupons and put them in order of what the best ones were, and what food we needed for the week. Later in the day, we would go food shopping.

My mom had a couple of credit cards, but she didn't want to use them, preferring instead to redeem the coupons we had meticulously cut out and saved. I could tell she was really embarrassed. You always notice the people at a store who only have coupons. It's a sure sign that they are poor.

She told me a story about us using those coupons and how I tried to cover for her. She said, "John, you did a really cute thing that day. When we were checking out, and you saw me reach for my stack of coupons, you said in a loud voice, so the cashier couldn't help but hear, 'Charge it.' I know you did that because you wanted to let the cashier know that we weren't poor and could use the credit cards if we wanted. That put a smile on my face."

So why tell you all this, for starters? To understand someone's personality, you need to know their history. Mine began in chaos.

TWO

JUST A SPERM DONOR

DESPITE THE ALMOST CONSTANT TURMOIL OF MY CHILDHOOD, I KNOW deep down my mom did the best she could. When I was a young kid, I realized it was very hard for her financially. When we were at the women's shelter, it was awful. The one thing that I clearly remember during those years was that I had to use powdered milk instead of the real stuff for my cereal. It was disgusting. My mom was working her butt off to get us out of the shelter, but it was always a struggle. One Christmas, I remember how excited I was to open my present, only to find a blanket, rather than the toy truck I dreamed about. I was heartbroken. When one of my friends told me that he got a PlayStation, I couldn't tell him the truth that all I got was a blanket. But I understood that my mom couldn't afford to buy me anything more expensive, so I laughed and pretended to be happy. I wouldn't betray her.

I also remember going with my mom to the local food pantry to get free stuff. She would take me every week to make sure I had enough food to keep me healthy. But she was too proud just to take the food and do nothing to give something back. Every time we picked up the food, we had to do some volunteer work at the shelter. We would help serve meals to the homeless, clean up the kitchen, or do whatever else they needed. I think that was the beginning of my understanding of what the "Golden Rule" really meant in practical terms.

She did a lot of nice things for me, too, which stuck with me somehow. For example, she arranged for a Big Brother for me from that organization,

8

and she got me into the Cub Scouts. But teaching me—showing me over and over—to help people was a lesson that stuck in my head far more than anything I learned in the Scouts or from any Big Brother.

I probably didn't realize it at the time, but I was also picking up quite a bit from my mom's brother, Uncle Toby Piper. Uncle Toby was a big man, over six feet tall and at least 250 pounds. He was an ex-Marine, although he was dishonorably discharged. The cause was likely the alcohol and drug problems he would face his entire life. Uncle Toby died at an early age, in fact, from an overdose of fentanyl. Despite all of that, I worshiped the man. He was always there for me and was the closest thing to a father I have ever had.

And he never seemed to be drunk or on drugs when I was around. I think he really had a soft spot for me. When we'd have Thanksgiving or Christmas dinner over at my grandparents' farmhouse, it was always Uncle Toby who took me out to the backyard to throw the football. I looked up to him. While he never seemed able to hold a job very long, he could do many practical things like change out a car's water pump and fix the many car problems we always seemed to have. He was also very handy around the house, and to me he was a hero on the home front. To a kid my age, that was impressive. Looking back, Uncle Toby *was* my father figure. I can still remember the trademark smirk that passed for his smile.

Even with Uncle Toby around, though, my mom had not given up on the idea of a real father for me. When I was about nine, she asked me if I wanted to reconnect with my biological dad, Mike. Looking back, I realize I probably had a powerful need for a real father; I think a lot of boys raised by single mothers have the same urge. She said that if she could find him, would I want to have a relationship with him, or just ask him for the child support he never paid? Of course, I did. Want a relationship, that is.

My mom decided to put an ad in a local paper in Texas, where she suspected he still lived. She actually got a response and was able to track him down. The ad said something like: "Looking for a man named Mike who lives in Cooper's Cove, Texas, and may be a U.S. Marine." As luck would have it, Mike's wife's cousin saw the ad and called Mike's wife, and she called my mom right away. They talked for a couple of hours. The woman told her that she would speak with Mike and ask if he wanted to connect with me. Apparently, he did.

I don't remember what Mike said to me on that phone call. All I remember is that I was so happy to hear his voice. Maybe, at long last, I would finally have a real dad, like other kids I knew. After only a couple of weeks, and much to my delight, Mike and his wife asked if I could come for a visit where they lived in Texas. That August, they bought me a one-way plane ticket, and off I went.

Their initial plan was for me to stay with Mike and his wife in Texas for six months so my mom could finish getting the degree she was working on. But they also told my mom and me that I could live with them even longer if things worked out. At the time, my mom was attending college to become a certified medical assistant, plus working a full-time job. But during her breaks from college, she made the long drive from Illinois to Texas to bring me some things I wanted, like my bike or other stuff she couldn't carry on a plane.

I'm not sure why—maybe a TBI gap, or the fact that it ended so badly—but I don't have vivid memories of that visit with Mike. I can't even remember what he looked like, or how he smelled or behaved. Yes, he would take me fishing and do all that other father/son stuff that I was missing. But mostly what I remember was the problems. I recall that there was a good amount of fighting between Mike and his wife; looking back, I'm sure most of it had to do with me. I was old enough to know this wasn't good.

I must have been there for only a couple of months, I'm not sure, when my mom arrived with my bike. I was so excited. But the night before my mom was ready to leave Texas and head back to Illinois, Mike's wife said to her, completely out of the blue: "Norma I think John needs to go home with you." My mom was flabbergasted. She couldn't fathom why. She figured Mike's wife didn't want me there anymore because they had a three-year-old son, and she was afraid I would drive a wedge between her kids and Mike. I was more than upset. The next morning, we packed our bags and left; I felt totally rejected.

After we returned to Illinois, I was really hurting. Even though I was so young, I vividly remember how my heart was broken and couldn't understand why Mike didn't want me anymore. Rejection is one of the most damaging things that can happen to anyone, let alone a young, impressionable child. Imagine looking forward to finally having a father figure in your life, then having your father want nothing to do with you. It cut me to the bone. Shattered my innocence. I went from a relatively happy child to an angry young man. And that change in my behavior was obvious to everyone around me, especially my mom. I would disobey her at times and was generally becoming sullen and depressed. Now, as an adult, I cannot imagine how someone can break the heart of a little boy. To get his hopes up, then have them crashing down. To give him stability and hope, then slash those dreams into pieces. For what? But that's what Mike did to me.

In the years to come, Mike's abandonment of me would transform my already chaotic childhood into an angry adolescent nightmare, as you'll see. And as an adult, it probably factored into my dogged determination to stay in the Marines after my first blast and the TBI. No way I would lose the Corps, too.

Eventually, my mom told me that Mike sent us a measly $50 a month for five months; after that, we never heard from him again. That was, until I was blown up the second time. He sent my mom an email out of the blue telling me in no uncertain terms what I should be doing after I was injured. Things like how I should be taking care of my wounds, dealing with the VA—stuff like that. What balls that guy had! My mom asked me if I wanted to respond. I said, "No, but you can if you want." She wrote back to him and simply said: "Thanks, but I've managed to take care of my son all these years alone and in his best interest."

I guess Mike was right after all. He was nothing more than a sperm donor.

THREE

MY ANGRY ADOLESCENCE

MY TENTH BIRTHDAY WAS SPENT AT MIKE'S HOUSE IN TEXAS. AFTER THAT crushing experience, my mom and I returned to our house in Rockford, Illinois. After a few days, Mike called to talk to me. He also sent a few letters. Since my mom worked two jobs, she relied on me to get the mail every day and put it on the kitchen table until she got home. One day, I noticed there was a letter from Mike. I opened it. This time, instead of sending fifty dollars, he said he wouldn't be getting in touch with me anymore or sending any more money.

At ten years old, I couldn't comprehend what that meant. I asked my mom to read the letter and explain it to me. She turned red and bit her lip as she read. Then she put the letter down and didn't say anything for what seemed like a long time. Finally, she turned to me: "John, don't worry. I'm here, and we'll get through this." I started bawling. I know she never wanted to prejudice me against Mike. She hoped that as I got older, I would make those decisions for myself. That took a lot for her, since she was clearly infuriated with Mike's behavior, not to mention his lack of financial support. She told me when I was a little older that her heart broke for me, because she saw I was hurting and couldn't understand how somebody could do that to a child. But she honored her rule never to talk trash about Mike in front of me.

For some reason, my recollections from this part of my childhood, before I started acting out, are really vague. Whether it's the trauma of the rejection—that part I don't have as much trouble remembering—or my brain injury, I can't say. Typically, older memories can be the hardest to recover. I will say that for someone like me, someone who had almost total recall of everything, a TBI can be incredibly frustrating, though not to the point of smashing your head into a wall or anything. Some guys do that. Fortunately, I don't. With me it's more like I want to stop, regroup a second, and try to remember my train of thought. I can't always do it, but I don't want help. I want to do it myself.

Sometimes, when I'm around strangers, they take my pauses as a sign of stupidity. It doesn't bother me that much. Still, the bottom line is that to lose so many of your memories—the things that make you who you are—well, that's something I wouldn't wish on anyone. That is one of the many challenges of having a traumatic brain injury. You forget things, have trouble with simple tasks, and your impulse control is not what it used to be. And the worst part is not remembering how to do your job, what you ate for dinner, and even who your spouse is. And as you'll see, it happens to me a lot.

Fortunately, I always had my mom there to help me. And as she and I much later discussed how Mike's abandonment affected me as a child, I was not terribly surprised to hear her tell me about how it changed my personality. I went from a sweet kid to a terror, she said. I was acting out at school. Making wisecracks in class. Not following directions and generally not getting along well with my classmates. I was that kid who was always getting in fights, too, sometimes at the drop of a hat. Anything would set me off. It could be a verbal slight or someone just calling me a name. My anger was raging, and my mom told me during that time that she was literally at her wits' end.

And that wasn't the worst of it. I also did something that to this day really bothers me. I began to steal money from my mom. First, it was a small amount, maybe a total of ten or fifteen dollars. I would sneak into her bedroom, where she had the rolls of quarters tucked away in her purse. I'm not sure how much I stole or what the motivation was. I guess it was for the thrill, or maybe I was hoping to get caught, but it was certainly a reckless and selfish thing to do. I spent the money on nonsense—candy, bubble gum, junk like that.

Of course, my mom caught on quickly to what I was doing. Back then, it seemed like she was always angry with me, always disappointed. I don't blame her because, as she recalled, I was out of control. I wouldn't listen to her, I talked back, and I was always looking for trouble. I was doing really crazy things like setting small fires in the basement of our house. (I always put them out; I wasn't quite ready to torch the whole house.) I was always doing the opposite of what she asked of me. If she wanted me to make my bed, I didn't. If she asked me to mow the lawn, I wouldn't. There were many times when she punished me, but it didn't matter.

And as if the fights, theft, and petty arsons weren't enough, I also ran away from home a lot. Usually, it was only for a day or two. I never once stopped to think about what was motivating me to behave that way, or the effect it had on my mom. I just wanted to lash out, and there seemed to be nothing my mom or anyone could do to stop it.

But that changed when I ran away from home for a solid week when I was fourteen. It may not surprise you to know I went to Uncle Toby's. He called my mom and told her not to worry, that I would be staying with him for a couple of days. Like I said, Uncle Toby always seemed to have my back.

I was still a mass of anger, and I had no idea why I was acting out. Looking back, it was obvious that I never got over Mike rejecting me in such a heartless manner. The scars, while not visible, were there for me in spades. I was always in mental turmoil. Thinking negative thoughts about who I was at the core. Was I worthy as a person? Would I ever amount to anything other than a mess of a human being? These were not the thoughts of a well-adjusted young man, for sure. And why else would I have been so nasty to my mom, rejected all convention, and chosen to be the bad boy at home and school?

But that little "break," it turned out, would change things. Because while I was staying at Uncle Toby's, despite his assurances, my mom called the police to report me missing.

When I returned, I learned that she had decided to teach me a hard lesson. She told one of the officers—a guy I had run into often during my bad years—about the fights, the fires, the thefts, the constant lip. She told him she was at the end of her rope and needed help. The officer told her that he didn't think taking me to juvenile detention was a good idea. He thought that I was basically a good kid, I guess. Along with my uncle, he was one of my rare allies back then. My mom disagreed. She told the officer: "Sir, I need some help with John. He's out of control, and I have to teach him a lesson. I think it's the only way John will ever be able to get it together."

So—and thanks, Mom—I ended up in court. My mom was called to the witness stand and told the judge, "Your honor, as you can see, my son needs help. He's been stealing money from me, getting in fights at school, and running away from home, sometimes for a week. I think he needs to learn a lesson, and I hope, your honor, you will help me turn his behavior around."

I guess the judge agreed. He ordered me to be sent to juvenile detention for one full week. I was handcuffed, booked, and fingerprinted, just like in the movies. That week in "juvey" was among the worst in my life. Juvey isn't hard time, there aren't rats in the cell or gang fights or anything, but it's awful for a kid. A lot of the meals were just a slice of bread, a piece of lunch meat, and a plastic envelope of mustard or ketchup. Nothing that could be used as a weapon. We got two hours a day to watch the communal TV and some exercise periods. But most of the time, I was in my cell, either reading or playing cards or a board game with my cellmate. But the confinement, the creeping sense that I might somehow be a criminal, scared the hell out of me. I'm sure that's what Mom had in mind.

I have to say, though, she was there for me during my incarceration. I remember she told me during one of her visits: "John, you can behave this way, act out all you want, but no matter what you do, I love you and you can't push me away." She also told me that the rules were the rules and I had to follow them if I didn't want to be going back.

A few days into my jail time, the judge apparently asked Mom if she wanted him to release me for Thanksgiving dinner with her. My mom, the ballbuster, said to him: "Your honor, leave him in for Thanksgiving. That way he'll learn what it's really like in prison for minors." That was pretty much the turning point for me. Scared straight, as they say.

The day after Thanksgiving my mom picked me up from juvenile detention. Before she could even put the key in the ignition, I turned to her and said: "Mom, I want to talk to you. I'm sorry, and I'm never going back there again. I'll never steal from you, I promise, and now I know right from wrong. I swear I'll never disobey you again." She asked me, "John, what made you change your mind?" I told her that aside from just being in jail, "The juvey's Thanksgiving dinner really sucked. It was nothing like yours, Mom. It was like getting food from the lunch line at school."

Yeah, like Dorothy said in *The Wizard of Oz*, "There's no place like home." (Oh, and by the way, I did eventually pay my mom back all the money—penny for penny—that I stole from her.)

Of course, she never mentioned to the court that her own punishments were no picnic, either. There was one time when she saw some burn marks and ashes on the basement floor. (Apparently, I had started one of my pathetic little pyrotechnics.) As she was going down the steps to investigate, she didn't realize I was a couple of steps above her. She suddenly turned and hit my right shoulder. I lost my balance and fell down the last few steps and ended up with some bruises on my back. And another time, after my mom caught me stealing, she whacked me with a spoon, and it left some bruises on my hands. When I went to school the next day, my teacher saw them, and soon the authorities arrived to remove me from our house. I was sent to live with my grandmother. Talk about abandonment: first Mike and now this?

My mom was only allowed to have supervised visits with me during this time. I'm sure it broke her heart, because she was trying to do the best she could as a single parent with an unruly child. And it was hard for me, too. Even though kids like me—the victims of neglect or abuse—constantly live in a state of fear, still the love between a parent and child is so strong that it keeps pulling us right back. That was certainly the case for me. I missed my mom. I can remember it was almost like Christmas when she came to visit.

Fortunately, this didn't last long. And I know Mom was desperately trying to make up for it all. She wanted to be a good mother and did everything she could to make amends. Once she saved up enough money to buy me a Hot Wheels set with all the tracks included; I was so excited. I think my mom was trying to be a responsible parent, and it sure didn't hurt that she showed her love with the most coveted toy in the world to me at the time.

Looking back, I know I've described a childhood out of a Charles Dickens novel. And remember, my erratic memory may have dredged up more negatives than positives. But there *were* a few positives, positives that would resonate in my life. Like the time my mom somehow got us hooked up with this guy who ran a farmer's market in Rockford. In the back of the market, there was a very small apartment, and that was where we lived for a while. This was after I lived at my grandmother's house. It took about a month or so, and my mom had to prove to the authorities that she could be a good parent. My mom would go to work and leave me with a list of things to do after school like cleanups, painting, fixing holes—that kind of stuff.

She also left me food, but it wasn't great: cheap mac 'n' cheese, noodles, things like that. I quickly got sick of it. So, I started making my own meals, using some of the farmers' market food. I made a pretty good spaghetti sauce, as I recall. Really, I think that was when the idea of becoming a chef occurred to me. When I started cooking my own food, I realized I was pretty good. I remember loving mac and cheese—who doesn't?—and mixing in different ingredients like tomatoes to make it more interesting. I felt great being able to create a meal, and my mom and I would even cook together when she wasn't at work. Those were some of the happy times I like to remember.

Why? Maybe it was because I became aware that I had some talent to do *something*. I don't recall if I had self-confidence back then—maybe not, from the shock of Mike and Adam's abuse—but I do recall a definite sense of accomplishment, a sense I was pretty damn good at something. It was a feeling I would get again a few years later in the Marines. Looking back, I know I was struggling. The hurt was so deep that I had to insulate myself from feeling vulnerable. And little victories like cooking fed my survival gene, giving me strength and determination to overcome all that would follow.

As I look back, my mom had her own challenges, and I give her credit for doing the best she could. She recognized my struggles and tried to help. For example, she arranged for me to see a psychiatrist to help me deal with my anger issues. I do remember the doctor asking me a bunch of questions, even though I'm not sure what they were and how I answered. I do recall thinking the whole thing was bogus, but I went along. I was diagnosed as having Attention Deficit Hyperactivity Disorder (ADHD), which explained my restlessness and my lack of attention to detail and following orders. And eventually, during those sessions, I began to open up and deal with my negative emotions. I remember every time the doctor brought up my dad, I would cry. I was surprised myself that I had bottled up all those emotions and that my negative behavior reflected that. You never get over a hurt like that. Never. But you do learn to cope.

My hellion days were finally over thanks to spending a week in juvey, going to see a psychiatrist, and finally realizing that my problems were not all my fault. I can also honestly say that my mom was a saint back then. She never gave up on me. She helped me understand something that to this day I still cherish: When life knocks you down, get up, dust yourself off, and move on. Never dwell on the loss.

Luckily, for me, there were better days ahead. I got into the school orchestra playing, of all things, the violin. It was the start of my love for music. Before long, I was the proud owner of a used, but beautiful, German violin. Incidentally, my mom researched the cost of the violin and saved almost enough money over the summer to buy it for me. When she came up a bit short, the owner let her pay the balance over another month. I took lessons and practiced regularly. My mom was still working two jobs, and she would call me and check in after school to make sure I had done my chores, practiced my violin, and completed all my homework.

I was very proud of my musical accomplishments. I moved up quickly in the orchestra—from the fourth to the second chair in only two years. On most nights when I got home from school, I would play a piece for my mom that I learned that day. And on one of her birthdays, I even planned a special surprise. I practiced the "Happy Birthday" song on my violin, and before she went to work, I went into her bedroom to play it for her. I had to restart twice but nailed it on the third try.

Around this time, my mom got me a small job—even though I was a kid—helping at a donut shop owned by her boyfriend. The reason I wanted to work was so that I could save up enough money to take my mom out to lunch for Mother's Day. It didn't pay much—a five-dollar bill here and there—but soon I had enough money to plan a superspecial Mother's Day outing.

I took this effort very seriously, almost with military precision. Here was my plan: first, I went into her closet and picked out the outfit I wanted her to wear; made sure I had enough cash to pay for her meal; and gave her the address of the restaurant where we were going. I never revealed my plan until we arrived. Of course, she drove us there, but I was really the one in the driver's seat, if you know what I mean.

"Mom, don't get out of the car," I said, as I hopped out of the passenger seat and went to her side of the car. I opened the door, gave her my arm, and off we went. I could see she was really surprised and happy but still unsure about what I was up to. As we walked to the entrance of the restaurant, I opened the door for her, and when the waitress led us to our table, I even pulled out her chair and helped her take off her sweater. She was shocked at this point. "Mom, I want to order your lunch. Would you like the cheeseburger and maybe a side salad to go with it?" Her eyes were as huge as golf balls, and she started to cry. I remember thinking, *I wonder why she's crying?* The cheeseburgers were awesome, and we had a great lunch. After we finished, the waitress brought over the check and placed it on the table in front of my mom. I slid the check over to my side of the table. *Wow,* I thought. *Didn't they realize I was the one going to pay, since the entire event was my idea?* I grabbed the check from the waitress and told her I was the one paying for the meal. Now the waitress's eyes were filling up with tears. *Oh no, here we go again,* I thought. I couldn't figure out what I did to make the waitress cry, but later that day my mom told me what the waitress said to her before we left. "Your little boy is so sweet. We were all so touched by him and what he did for you."

I must admit I felt great. Everyone was happy, most of all my mom.

I was also playing football, which enabled me to channel that excess energy I had and I'm sure on some level kept my anger in check. My mom did her best to attend my football games. But she was working two jobs, so she couldn't make it that often. In fact, most of the time, no one came to my football games at all. Often, when I would glance up to see if someone I knew was there, I was crushed that the stands were empty. There were times that I walked off the field when the game was over and cried. But I had my good moments, too. One day, we were practicing one of our drills. The coach put our team in a ring, created a circle, then would call on two people, one offensive and the other defensive. He called me first, then a guy who was bigger than me. The goal was for the defensive guy to take down the offensive guy. When the whistle blew, I exploded out of my stance, launched myself up and through my opponent, and put him down on his back. That victory was sweet!

I can truly say that music and sports, along with my mom's tough love, helped slay my adolescent demons. I also had Uncle Toby. In fact, my troubles seemed to bring us closer. He had two sons of his own, and I became the third. Many weekends we would just hang out. He would take us fishing and, later, cooked food we absolutely loved—and it always included lots of hot spice. Insanely hot, I might add. We had a lot in common. We both liked the outdoors, and we loved to cook and eat. Uncle Toby also gave me acceptance and respect. Uncle Toby meant so much to me that I would later create a special chili recipe just for him. Two whole habaneros were the ticket.

Lord knows Uncle Toby had his demons. But before he died, he got it together, found God, and turned his life around. I can honestly say he was my hero. I love spicy food to this day because of him. Uncle Toby was my emotional savior. I needed his comfort and advice, in the years to come. And sometimes that comfort came in strange and unexpected ways, as you'll see after that awful day in Afghanistan.

FOUR

The Young Buck Discovers the Marines

Bᴜᴛ ᴍʏ ʟɪꜰᴇ ɪɴ Rᴏᴄᴋꜰᴏʀᴅ ᴡᴏᴜʟᴅ ꜱᴏᴏɴ ᴄᴏᴍᴇ ᴛᴏ ᴀɴ ᴇɴᴅ ᴡʜᴇɴ ᴍʏ mom and her third husband, Gene, decided to move us to Antioch, Illinois.

Gene was huge—six feet two, and damn near 400 pounds. At first, I had high hopes for him. He seemed like a nice guy—light years from Adam. My mom started seeing him while he lived in Chicago and we were still in Rockford. She married him with the same optimism as I had. Hey, three's the charm, right? Gene's mom owned a three-story building in Chicago. Each story had enough room for an entire family. At some point, they grew tired of living in Chicago, so Gene's mom decided to sell the house. She divided the proceeds among her children. Gene and my mom decided to buy a house in Antioch, Illinois, which I now consider my hometown.

I should say a word about Antioch here, since the folks there have been great to me in the years since. Antioch is roughly sixty miles north of Chicago, right up by Lake Michigan and the Wisconsin border. (It has nothing to do with Antioch College, by the way, which is in Ohio.) The last time they did a census was in 2010, and I think it said that only 14,430 people were living there. I believe the entire town is only about eight-and-a-half square miles, so everybody knew what their neighbors were up to, which for me wasn't always so good.

Most of the people that lived there were what I would call lower middle class, except for a few professional types. But the town had heart. In my youth, I never realized how special the people in Antioch were. But later in my life, the good folks of Antioch would rally around me when I was going through a painful divorce and trying to cope with losing all four of my limbs.

We found a nice house in Antioch, and it was Gene, Mom, me, and his two daughters who would be living there. Because the house only had three bedrooms and there were five of us, Gene started building bedrooms in the basement for his eldest daughter and me. It was weird at first, but Gene made the basement arrangement work. He framed the room out, took some fabric panels and hung them up on each side of the room by two-by-fours. That gave us privacy.

I have to say, Gene was cool at first. He seemed to like me, and I could see he was trying to make the best of what was probably for him a big adjustment. I'm sure for him I was a handful. (Despite my "juvey" revelation, I was still no choir boy.) The more we lived together, the more he seemed hell-bent on controlling me. Hey, I wasn't his son, but he sure acted like I was. Being an adolescent, and coming from the troubled background I came from, having someone tell me what to do, where to go, and what to wear—well, let's just say it wasn't working for me.

By my senior year in high school, me a young, eighteen-year-old buck, I had really begun to chafe under the rules that Gene and my mom had laid down. But there wasn't much I could do. I dared not confront Gene. Remember, he was a 400-pound behemoth, and I was a skinny teen. Thank God he wasn't out of the Adam mold. His punishments mostly ran to grounding me, and, I must admit, he treated me as fairly as his own kids. Still, there was tension.

Things were better at school, though. When we moved to Antioch, it was too late to play football, and they didn't have an orchestra. So, instead, I took photography lessons at school. I loved it. We got to play with the old-school cameras that you manually adjust for things like shutter speed and light. I remember I got an A-plus for a photo I took of, of all things, a flower. The wildflower was growing behind our house, where a ravine connected the back of our house to our neighbor's. I took a photo of it in focus, and a few more out of focus. It made for a very interesting image.

I also joined our high school choir. I was making some great friends in the process and beginning to feel that I belonged. I wish I could remember all of their names but having the TBI can often block out some of the most important people in your life, and this was certainly the case here. However, I do recall that having these new friends gave me a real sense of accomplishment. That I was important, competent, and accepted. I loved being part of that group as well, and I developed some strong friendships. I also began to feel much better about myself. As my accomplishments grew, so did my self-confidence. I was now being rewarded by positive experiences, and not punished for negative ones. I felt at that time that there was hope. That despite all the crap I had to deal with most of my life, there was a light at the end of the tunnel. A ray of sunshine. A song. A flower. And a new job.

I started working at the McDonald's in Antioch, which was great because finally I made some money. But I soon got suspended for falling asleep at the drive-thru window. The funny thing was, I thought they were going to fire me, so I quit. Then, I found out that they weren't going to fire me at all, but just suspend me to teach me a lesson. But I had already made up my mind to leave. I was stubborn as a mule back then.

At some point, Mom and Gene told me that they wanted me to pay rent, which wasn't so bad, but they also told me I had to be home at ten o'clock every night. An eighteen-year-old guy with a ten o'clock curfew? Are you kidding me? So that summer I decided to move out.

Now it was just me and Rascal, a fox rat terrier I got when I was sixteen. I should mention that I'm almost never without a dog. I have always loved animals, and they would play a significant role in my life, especially after I was injured. Rascal started it all. Like me, he was headstrong, restless, and intelligent. So, there was no way I would leave my best friend behind when I decided to go out on my own. I guess I love dogs so much because they are loyal to a fault. No matter what you do, they are always there for you. Rascal and I lived in my old beat-up car for two weeks, near my friend Kevin's house. It was uncomfortable sleeping in a small vehicle with only two doors. To try to get some sleep, I would put the driver's seat down all the way. But being a six-footer at this point, nothing really helped that much. Rascal and I had many sleepless nights in that car.

In the meantime, I got a job at a Renaissance Fair, where I helped kids climb up on the rock walls—the ones with the little plastic footholds. Some days I struggled because I was so tired from tossing and turning in the car. But it was always better on hot days when Rascal came with me, and we hung out together behind one of the walls in the shade. (On cool days, I would sometimes leave him in the car.) At least I had my buddy with me.

Looking back, my life was crazy. Here I was with no real direction, living in a car with my dog. I had just enough money to buy dog food for Rascal; I ate the free food at my job. At one point, I moved in with a buddy of mine and his family, which was a brief moment of stability. His parents were great—they even offered to send me to culinary school. But I just didn't feel right about that. I thanked them, but I had to do stuff on my own. I moved out, still without a plan for my life.

I know by that age a lot of kids—boys and girls—have some kind of future in mind. I really didn't. Maybe it was all the pain I suffered as a child, maybe my brain was just too preoccupied with all the bad stuff rattling around. But somewhere in my head were some vague thoughts about becoming a soldier, like my superpatriotic Army mom or a Marine like my Uncle Toby. Or maybe 9/11 hit me harder than I thought.

The attack happened two days before my fifteenth birthday, and, like older people with the shooting of President Kennedy, I remember it vividly. I was sitting in my school auto CAD (computer-assisted drawing) class when my teacher heard about what happened and turned on the television. I watched in disbelief as the second airplane crashed into one of the Twin Towers. I was literally sick to my stomach when both toppled to the ground; I couldn't fathom the whole thing. My mom tried to explain it to me later that day, but nothing she said made me feel better. What made it worse was that my mom told me someone she knew had a friend who was killed in the Pentagon that day.

And who knows? Maybe it was watching that gruesome scene on television in school that may have subconsciously lit a fire under me. Maybe somewhere in the back of my head, I sort of knew I wanted to join the military and take out those vile terrorists! But even after witnessing the terrorist attack while it was happening, I didn't dwell on it during the following weeks. I had a lot going on in my high school years. Sadly, now because of my traumatic brain injury, I can't recall much of that period of my life, except for moments like 9/11, which, despite my TBI, I could never completely forget.

So, there I was, fresh out of high school with no clue about much of anything, let alone what I wanted to do with my life. In that time between high school and the Marines, a period of some fifteen months, I hung out around Antioch, killing time and taking some odd jobs like the ones I mentioned. None of the jobs meant anything to me other than a few bucks.

Except for one. I took a job at an Old Navy store near the Gurnee Mills Mall, a huge shopping center near Antioch and the Great Lakes Naval Base on Lake Michigan. At the time, I recall I was still shy around girls, although I was interested in one girl. But to my surprise, this girl told me that another girl working at Old Navy, a really cute brunette named Darlene, had eyes for me. She told me that Darlene wanted me to go to a party with her.

I did, and in short order, we began going out. I liked her smile and the way she looked at me. Over the course of a few months, we grew a lot closer, and, yes, in my teenage mind, romance had flowered. In fact, I began thinking we would be husband and wife someday. There was a catch, though. Her parents didn't like me. They thought I had no idea what I wanted to do with my life. (Which was true.)

I believe it was around then when it occurred to me that maybe I should think about joining the military. After all, you want your girlfriend to think you're headed *somewhere*, and a lot of girls that age really dig young, tough military guys. I remembered how strongly I felt after 9/11, and now being two years older, I decided to make a visit to interview with a few recruiters—just like my mom did when she was my age. After all, the military was in my family, even though Uncle Toby's Marine career didn't end so well. I decided to give it a try.

What I really wanted was to be a fighter pilot. I had a meeting with the Navy recruiter, and he told me in no uncertain terms, "Mr. Peck, you are just too tall to fit in the cockpit." I met with an Army guy, too, but I really don't remember what he said. But the guy I clearly remember was the Marine recruiter, a Sgt. White. For some reason, he made an impression on me. Maybe it was the uniform.

In those days, the recruiters were all located in offices near one another in this strip mall near where we lived. I recall waiting with my mom outside the Navy's guy's office, and luckily for me, Marine Sgt. White spotted us and called us over. He was very encouraging. A colleague of his, a master gunnery sergeant, also interviewed me, and he told me he saw me as more of an infantry guy, maybe even a squad leader. This guy delivered a great sales job. I asked my mom what she thought about his pitch, and she was very impressed. In fact, he was so persuasive that right on the spot I told him, "Sign me up!"

And, with that, my life was changed forever. The Marines would teach me the truth about the old saying: what doesn't kill you makes you stronger.

FIVE

Becoming a Marine

MOM HELD A GOING-AWAY PARTY FOR ME A FEW DAYS BEFORE MY IN-duction. It was her and Gene, his daughters, and my grandparents. There wasn't any drinking, but it got silly anyway. At one point, I took some electric clippers and gave myself a reverse mohawk—that is, shearing off a three-inch runway right down the middle of my scalp, leaving the sides like a circus clown. Then I inhaled helium from the balloons, talking like Donald Duck until my lips turned blue and I almost passed out.

I was all business, though, on September 11, 2005, two days before my twentieth birthday and on the fourth anniversary of 9/11. My mom drove me to Chicago, where I would meet the other Marine recruits before flying to California to begin our basic training. It was about an hour-and-a-half ride, and to be honest, I was glad she was with me. Once we got to where I was to report, my mom dropped me off, and that was that. I was going to be a United States Marine.

I checked in with Sgt. White, who warned me not to drink and to behave myself. On the drive in, I noticed that were lots of girls around, and no lack of bars. But despite the temptations, I took the sergeant's advice and behaved. I spent the night alone in a hotel—very excited and anxious. I may have tried to watch television; I can't remember. The next morning, I took an early plane bound for San Diego. I remember how beautiful it looked landing in San Diego, the sparkling Pacific Ocean to the west and the San Diego Bay and city skyline to the east. But once we deplaned, it was all business. I boarded a bus, along with about thirty other superamped recruits, for the short drive to the Marine Corps Recruit Depot (the MCRD, in Marine lingo), which was basically next door.

When the bus pulled up, for a second, it was quiet. I remember idly watching a plane take off at the airport. Then all hell broke loose. I don't know how many of you have experienced military boot camp, but with the Marines, it's 24/7 balls-out intense from the instant the bus arrives at the depot. A Marine drill instructor (DI) hopped on the bus and, neck veins bulging, screamed, "From now on, you answer 'Aye, Aye, Sir' to anything I say! Do you understand?"

I yelled, "Aye, Aye, Sir" as loud as I could. And so began my Marine Corps training.

At the time, sectarian violence was building in Iraq in the wake of the U.S. invasion, and thousands of Marines were already in the country. Even recruits like me had a sense that they would be sent into combat. Still, nothing can prepare you for the insanity of the first two hours of Marine boot camp.

With several drill instructors (DIs) serenading us at high decibels, our motley little group of about thirty recruits was herded into formation, our feet positioned over the famous yellow footsteps that every Marine who did boot camp in San Diego well remembers. If you're a second slow, the DIs instantly swoop in and threaten to burst your eardrums.

Under this constant harassment, we learned how to stand at attention. Of course, I knew how to do that already. My mom was at heart a drill instructor. We were told we were no longer covered by the U.S. Constitution. Kind of ominous. As members of the U.S. military, Constitutional rights are suppressed; you are instead now subject to military law, as laid out in the Uniform Code of Military Justice (UCMJ). The penalties for breaking this code—going AWOL or disobeying an order, for example—are severe. Trust me, you do *not* want to end up in a Marine Brig.

Then we were rushed into a room and told to stand in front of these waist-high red desks, clutching what few personal things we had tightly to our chests.

"Everything out! Empty your pockets!" the instructors yelled at us and went down the line, stopping every so often to single out some poor laggard, to search for anything contraband—knives, porn, drugs, condoms, etc. Letters from wives, girlfriends, and moms were thrown on the floor. All we could keep were any religious things—bibles, what have you—and our contact information.

All this goes into a white mesh bag that we threw over our left shoulders. (A couple of guys slung it over their right shoulders and were immediately doubled-teamed by the DIs.) Our cell phones, wallets, everything else we brought were taken—not to be returned until a few days before graduation.

We were then herded into the next room for our only phone call for the next eleven weeks. As the DIs continued shouting, we lined up. I remember barely being able to think. Right beside the phone was a sign telling us what to say and *only* what to say: "I'm in Marine Corps Recruit Depot in San Diego. The next time I contact you will be by mail in two to three weeks. I'm okay, I love you, goodbye." When it was my turn, I called my mom, recited this and only this to her, hung up, and jumped right back in line. Then they shuffled us over to the barbers. These guys are pros. They can turn the hairiest hipster bald in four or five quick strokes. And they seemed to enjoy the humiliation. No gashes, but several guys came out with bloody nicks and scrapes. Not me, though. My head was already as smooth as a cue ball.

Still in civilian clothes, we were lined up in what will become our platoon, which is part of a larger company. We met our new DI, along with two other Marine sergeants. These three men would be our personal guides through twelve weeks of incredibly demanding training. They would teach us to become models of honor, integrity, and—oh yes—highly efficient killers.

But once we got our uniforms and the initial shock of our "welcome" wore off, our days began to fall into a pattern. We were awakened each day at four in the morning by screaming DIs; sometimes they banged trash cans near our heads. We raced to the bathroom—now called "the head"—to shave and brush our teeth. Then it was straight to the mess hall for breakfast.

Eating as a Marine recruit is a unique and jarring experience. The food they give you is standard stuff—eggs, omelets, bacon for breakfast; sandwiches for lunch; meat and potatoes for dinner. (And there was even real milk instead of the nasty powdered milk I had to eat in my cereal as a kid.) But now, instead of eating alone, you eat as a platoon. That is, the first guy gets his plate, then stands at the table until the entire platoon is served. Then the DI shouts, "Sit." We sit as a group, and he yells, "Eat!" Even then, they give you only around fifteen minutes. So, the game is stuff as much food in your mouth as possible within that time limit. What was worse, we got no dessert until the last phase of training. No surprise that I dropped twenty pounds in boot camp.

I learned very quickly that the DIs loved to play mind games with you. They wanted people to fuck up, so they could scream at them and make them examples of what *not* to do. I also learned not to have my mom ship me candy or anything, for that matter, with the Marine insignia or *Semper Fidelis* (the Corps motto, usually shortened to *Semper Fi*). The candy they would immediately throw away; anything close to Marine markings on packaging would get you ridiculed at ear-splitting volume for being unworthy as yet for the title of U.S. Marine.

There were benefits, of course. First among them was a shift in thinking by Darlene's parents. I now had a career, and a macho one at that. I also managed to achieve some status within the platoon. Because at one point I was a lifeguard at Six Flags, I became the unit's "witch doctor," a title that involved helping my mates with minor medical stuff like foot blisters. (Moleskin is great, by the way.) And despite everything, the DIs never quite knocked the stubbornness out of me—a fact that made me proud. For example, I still referred to myself as "I" sometimes when answering my DIs. That's not good. Recruits are only allowed to refer to themselves as "this recruit." But I did it anyway.

Marine basic training is highly structured and broken down into three phases. Phase One introduced us to our rifles—the M16 from the Vietnam era. It can fire a 5.56 mm round with an effective range of 600 yards. I loved it. We were taught basic first aid, Marine history, and how to prepare for inspections. As you would expect, there's tons of physical challenges— long runs, sprints, learning to strike enemies, bayonet them, smash them with rifle butts, and cut them with knives. We even had a martial arts program, where our DIs showed us some basic moves. Then they put us in a pit with boxing gloves and mouthguards and made us fight against each other for three minutes. I held my own, but those three minutes felt much longer.

Two of my favorite exercises were the pugil sticks and the obstacle course. Pugil sticks are rods with big pads on both ends. Wearing a helmet and flak jacket, you fight another recruit; think Robin Hood and Little John fighting with staffs on a log. I wasn't a beast, but again I held my own. But I really loved the obstacle course. I still remember the recommended move to go over the top on the high wall. I aced it. And swim week was cool, too, or so I heard. They taught you how to jump off a ship—arms crossed and tight, feet together to protect your balls when you hit the water. You also have to jump in a pool and swim in full uniform, boots included. I did none of this, though, having come down with pneumonia. But I recovered quickly, just in time for Phase Two.

Phase One is the most challenging physically, but Phase Two ramps it up in terms of actual combat training. Field maneuvers get closer to simulating combat patrols and missions. You crawl under barbed wire in the mud, with blank rounds blasting all around. You crawl in ankle-deep water, shells going off nearby. But, and I loved this, you spend a lot of time on the rifle range. I was either "in the pit," laughing and joking with my buds while we changed targets or being taught how to shoot my weapon on the firing line. I did well. I was a sharpshooter. Only "expert" is better.

Ah, but the shit really hits the fan in Phase Three. That included weeks eight through twelve, then graduation. This was the final stretch. Hikes now went seven miles. We learned how to rappel down walls. We were led into a gas chamber and actually gassed, but not with anything lethal. It's all about getting you confident using your gas mask, but it can be tricky. Several guys in my platoon freaked out. The gas truly does burn your eyes, and it is seriously scary.

The real nut-cutter, though, is what they called, "the crucible." This is where you find out whether you're a Marine or not. We were bused north to the Camp Pendleton Marine Base, an enormous 122,798-acre site facing the Pacific Ocean between San Diego and Los Angeles. It's a grueling fifty-four hours of intense maneuvers, and we were down to two rations a day and maybe three hours of sleep. The pressure is tremendous. Even the DIs get tense.

The culmination of the crucible is this steep mountain called "The Reaper." You gotta go up it humping maybe seventy pounds of gear on your back. It was so bad that I had to push down hard on my knees to get the momentum to keep climbing. The DIs struggled, too. But, sweating gallons, my heart pounding, I made it! I still remember the rush, the pride I felt at completing the toughest physical challenge of my life. But mostly I remember just wanting to sleep. I was exhausted and close to my breaking point. But I was a finally a United States Marine!

I remember graduation day clearly. My mom came out to San Diego. Me and the guys I was training with spent the day getting our uniforms ready, making sure even the edges of our dress shoes sparkled. Then we put on our green t-shirts and shorts and did a three-mile run around the whole recruit depot. They announced over loudspeakers to the visitors that the Marines were heading back to their barracks to get ready for the ceremony. We showered and dressed in green trousers, khaki shirts, and our pointed cloth caps sometimes referred to as "piss cutters." As you probably have guessed, there's a salty Marine nickname for damn near everything.

The crowning moment of the ceremony was getting our EGAs—the coveted eagle, globe, and anchor insignias that mark us as true U.S. Marines. When it was my turn, I took the EGA from my staff sergeant, shook his hand, and stood back in line. When all of us received our EGAs, the captain ended the event and dismissed us. We yelled the Marine chant, "Ooo-rah!" I may have yelled louder than most. Now I belonged. Now I had really done *something*.

After our dismissal, the pressure was off. We strolled around the base with our guests, in my case, my mom. And we could even chat normally with the same DIs who screamed insults at us for the past three months. We got to ask them what they got their ribbons for, which was kind of a great way to see what lay ahead. It's cool; we were all in the Corps now.

One of our DIs cautioned me about going out and eating greasy fast food right away; we'd been on a pretty good diet for these twelve weeks. So, what was the first thing I did after it was all over? I went to a McDonald's, where I was never officially fired, and ordered a double cheeseburger and fries anyway. And, yeah, I paid the price, if you know what I mean. After I recovered, that night we officially got our orders. Like I signed up for, I was being sent to the school of infantry (SOI) in Camp Pendleton.

I graduated right around the Christmas break, so I got a week off. I decided to go home to Illinois for a brief visit. Darlene and I had been communicating by phone or writing letters to each other, but as a recruit I didn't have time to see her in person, and besides, I was totally focused on my training.

Like I said before, the store where Darlene and I met was near the Navy's Great Lakes base, where Navy folks do their basic training. So there were always lots of Navy folks, men and women, walking around like they were really something. It used to piss me off. The first thing I did when I got back home was put on my full-dress Marine uniform—blue trousers, navy jacket with gold buttons, a snow-white belt and hat, or cover, as they say in the Corps. It's the best uniform in the military, bar none. We call it the "panty dropper."

I drove to the mall, got out of the car I borrowed from my mom, and walked in with my new Marine swagger. You bet I got some serious looks that day, too. The first thing I did was pass by that clothing store, and as I walked by, I could see my reflection in the store window. I looked damn good. Now, those same jerks who thought they were something were nothing compared to me. They would never be able to go through what I just did. That's why being a Marine is the best.

That singular moment made me realize that despite having had a rough childhood and experiencing loss, pain, and abuse—I was a survivor. There was something in my DNA that kept me bobbing up in the ocean rather than drowning. Just like my mom and Uncle Toby. But, whatever it was, I began to believe I was the luckiest guy in the world. I could have never imagined at that point in time that my luck wouldn't last.

SIX

REFINING MY SKILLS

HE U.S. MARINES—LIKE NAVY SEALS AND DELTA GUYS—ARE OFTEN THE "tip of the spear," military talk for the first units sent on extremely dangerous missions. After boot camp, new Marines are sent to advanced training to learn the specific combat skills that make them part of that spear.

In my case, it was the School of Infantry (SOI). So, after a few days back home, it was off to Camp Pendleton. The School of Infantry turns Marines who are straight out of boot camp into combat-ready Marines. It's more relaxed than boot camp. You still have to greet those who outrank you, but no one's in your face screaming. The instructors are more like teachers. In five weeks, they turn you into an expert on one of the many weapons Marines use—like machine guns and antitank rockets. In my case, it would be the mortar.

The 81mm mortar, a weapon I would become very familiar with, is a skinny metal tube that can throw a ten-pound shell in a high arc over 5,000 meters. It's a stone-cold killer from above. On impact, a high-explosive shell can kill anyone within thirty-to-forty meters and throw body-shredding hot metal shrapnel even further. It can also fire shells that explode high up and illuminate a target, and white phosphorus shells. The phosphorus shells are especially nasty. They can literally burn the flesh off your bones. But before I got intimately acquainted with my lethal new friend, there were problems.

For one thing, some of my boot camp buddies were also assigned to Pendleton. One was Ian Gilbert, a snuff-dipping twenty-one-year-old from Idaho. Gilbert was one of the coolest Marines I met, a low-key, sort of serious guy that everyone seemed to respect, even guys senior to him. There was also Martin Kelly, the complete opposite. Kelly was a total goofball, a Washington State kid who loved beer and loved to push the limits, not a great idea in the Marines. He got yelled at a lot, but he developed this "boot shrug"—hey, I'm a stupid boot. What did you expect?—that often let him skate by. But if you were ever down, Kelly was the guy who could cheer you up. These two were "my guys," and we would stay supertight.

At twenty-one, Ian could buy beer in California. Martin and I couldn't, but we were always thirsty, if you get my drift. All young guys have the potential to get into trouble. Double that for young hell-raising Marines.

Like there was this one time I wrapped a sheet around my head like a turban and ran into another barracks screaming, "Allah akbar, I'm gonna kill you motherfuckers." It was great. They were chasing me around, and I was running around yelling Arabic at the top of my lungs. But when I tried to race out, somebody grabbed me, pulled the sheet, and yanked me backward. Suddenly, I felt something warm running down my arm.

It turns out I had slashed my wrist crosswise on a steel plate near a light switch. There was blood everywhere. I started screaming. Someone put pressure on it, and they rushed me to the emergency room. It took sixteen stitches to sew me up.

That meant I would have to wait before joining a company for SOI training because pull-ups are part of the physical requirements. To kill time, they made me patrol the base. Martin Kelly and I discovered secret spots where one guy could nap, while the other guy stood lookout. But after a few days, despite having my wrist wrapped, I was able to pass the test and convince a sergeant to let me pick up with a company. There was no obstacle that could ever stop me from being a United States Marine.

Ian Gilbert, Martin Kelly, and I all got into mortar training. In addition to endless drills on the weapon, there were classroom sessions on maneuvers and physical requirements, including a 20K hike; PT never stops for a Marine. Still, I managed to step in it from time to time. One of our mortar instructors was this short little sergeant. He was really an okay guy, and he had only one rule: no snuff-dipping in his class. Well, I had already started to piss him off by never addressing him as sergeant, as in, "How do you do such and such," instead of, "Sergeant, how do you do such and such?" Then one day, he was instructing us during drills. I spit. He stopped. "Peck, what in the hell is in your mouth?" he shouted. "What is my one rule?" I yelled back, "I'm guilty. It's snuff." The other part of the rule is if you dip and get caught, you gotta swallow it. Turns out he was kidding about the swallowing part. But I did it before anyone could tell me otherwise. I didn't throw up, but I did get really dizzy. Not an experience I'd recommend.

During this time, I also got engaged to Darlene. She was not only a pretty girl, but someone I could talk to. Someone I could be myself with. Darlene was responsible, stable, and trustworthy. All of those qualities I needed in a woman. Most of all, I knew she loved me for the person I was and hoped to be. And now that I was an official Marine, I was hoping her parents would look at me as a person worthy of marrying their daughter.

Like I said, being a Marine had warmed her dad up, but her mom not so much. I think I really cemented my relationship with her dad on my first visit to their house when I was in boot camp. He and her brother were hanging drywall, and I volunteered to hold it up while they did the ceiling. Trust me; it wasn't easy.

Darlene and I talked on the phone a lot when I was at Pendleton, and she wrote to me all the time. I was impressed that even though I was in the military, and might have long stretches of duty overseas, Darlene seemed to have the stuff to stick with me. And when I closed my eyes, I could clearly see her face. I decided to ask her to marry me.

I finally worked up the courage to ask her dad for her hand in marriage over the phone. He broke down and cried. Then I asked Darlene, and she said "yes" right away. But right after that, she told me she wanted an engagement ring from Tiffany. I had no idea what Tiffany was but sure found out when I found the store's address in San Diego and decided to check out the rings. Let's put it this way: it's not Zales. So, $1,300 later, I left the store with a Tiffany diamond engagement ring. Despite to me what was a huge price tag, for Tiffany it was nothing. To me, the diamond looked like a grain of sand. I'm sure she hoped for a huge rock, but then again, she was going to marry a young, relatively broke, newly minted U.S. Marine.

After we got engaged, I completed SOI training. I was now ready for deployment. My graduation from SOI was anticlimactic. And a bit disappointing. It turned out that my mom couldn't afford to come to San Diego again. Darlene couldn't make it, either. And that night, I remember one guy getting his orders and finding out he had a month's break before reporting for duty. Me? My orders were the same as Ian's and Martin's. They were:

Third Battalion, First Marine Division, headquartered guess where. Camp Pendleton. The buses were right there waiting to take us over; there would be no break for me.

Our bus pulled up to the grinder (that's the parade ground for the battalion) and dropped us off. A lot of other guys were there too, waiting to get assigned. We arranged our gear in neat little piles and stood around. Before long, the battalion sergeant major came out and introduced himself.

I was assigned to an 81mm mortar platoon, as per my enlistment agreement. So were Gilbert, Kelly, and a kid named—no kidding—Alex Kielbasa. You can only imagine the abuse we heaped on Kielbasa.

Typically, this kind of platoon consists of eight mortars, each with a four-man team, for a total of thirty-two men. Each team consists of a squad leader, an ammo man, a gunner who puts the target info into the sight, and an assistant gunner who actually drops the shell down the tube. The ammo man has the worst job; he's gotta haul all the shells, which are heavy. I also got my permanent gear. Up until now, we had to return the gear we used. So, I now got my own M16, flak jacket, Kevlar cover (you'd call it a helmet) for both the desert and woods, main pack, and a camelback water container with a hose, for drinking on the go. I had my name sewn into all my new stuff. Yeah, I'd done some things before, but this made me feel great! This was *my* Marine gear. *I* did this.

During this period, I was living in a ratty little one-story barracks they called a flattop. I later learned ours was condemned for asbestos. Worse, we were constantly subjected to harassment by a group of young lance corporals. These guys had already been on deployment. They called themselves "senior" lance corporals, and they were determined to make us respect their rank. They often barged in at night, sometimes drunk, and made us do stuff like push-ups and going into the shower with our full gas kits on. And they made it clear that anyone who snitched would face "repercussions." We weren't sure what that meant, but nobody wanted to find out.

One night, they burst in and found out that one of us, a kid named Joe Houston, had a birthday. They grabbed the kid, bundled him into a car, and took off for Oceanside, a nearby beach town, to get him drunk. Well, they sure succeeded. In fact, when they dropped him off, he was so out of it that we were afraid he had alcohol poisoning. He didn't, but he sure as hell couldn't get up the next morning.

Our sergeants, of course, immediately noticed all this and began grilling us. The code was not to snitch, but Marine sergeants usually got what they wanted. Finally, Kielbasa caved. In short order, it seemed like every-body knew Kielbasa snitched. But it ended up helping me. Because not too long after, this lance corporal named Robinson came into our barracks and asked us to gather around. Now by this time, we were wise to their tricks. For example, when lance corporals came in and asked us, "Who wants ice cream?" it generally meant they were recruiting for a working party. But this guy sounded legit. First, he asked us: "How many of you guys are intelli-gent?" Well, Joe Houston, Kielbasa, and I slowly raised our hands. Then he said: "Keep your hands up if you scored better than 250 on the PT test." Now it was just Kielbasa and me. (I had a 279. I'll never forget that.) Then he said, "Kielbasa, you're out because you ratted."

He pulled me aside. "You are now a forward observer for a mortar pla-toon," he told me. "Peck, you still gotta listen to your sergeant, but you're with us FOs now."

Just what I wanted! A forward observer is the guy who ranges far ahead of the gun team and actually has eyes on the enemy. He calls in the location of the target and adjusts the fire until the target is hit. Robinson introduced me to the other FOs, and before long, I was out of the flattop and into a squad bay in a nice four-story building. I even got a two-man room. Of course, this being the Marines, not everything is easy street. In this build-ing, you have to "field day" your room. This means you take everything out of the room and thoroughly clean the empty room—floors, walls, ceilings. Then you clean all your stuff outside the room, then move it back. We did this every Thursday.

Also, there was the issue of my haircut. We got a haircut every week, and by now I was getting a medium regulation, courtesy of a friendly lance cor-poral, meaning the fade starts halfway up the side of my head. I could have at least some hair on top. This is opposed to the "high and tight," which basically shaved the side of your head and left a pathetic one-quarter inch on top. Some of the high and tighters resented my obviously cooler look.

Meanwhile, I was still talking to my fiancée and planning our wedding. So, I went to the platoon sergeant and told him I was getting married and would need some leave time. It's kind of unheard of for a new guy to be getting married this early in training. That's not to mention living off-base, which I would be allowed to do as a married man.

Still, even the Marines can't tell you not to get married. So, I left Pendleton for Illinois. Darlene and I were married in May 2005. We had a small wed-ding, just family really. Even though my TBI has blurred the memory, I still recognize it as one of the best days of my life. Having a new wife and a new and challenging career in the Marines took me in a different direction mentally—to a place where I longed to be for most of my troubled life. Fuck you, sperm donor Mike. Now the Marines want me; my wife wants me!

Darlene's parents paid for our honeymoon to Disney World in Orlando, Florida. But there was one hitch. They came with us! That was weird to me, and I wish I could say I liked the idea. But the truth was that I was too young to drink. Oh well. I guess I was so focused on my career in the Marines that I simply accepted this unconventional arrangement as a fact of life. Darlene's parents were actually very nice people, so it could have been much worse!

When the honeymoon was over, I headed back to Pendleton by myself. I spent my weekends looking for an apartment in Oceanside. Once I found one, Darlene would come out and we would live off-base. But until she arrived, I had plenty of training still ahead of me.

The training was very intense and specialized. I learned how to be a forward observer for a mortar team. This involved calling in coordinates and, of course, plenty of hiking—my strong suit. But, somehow, I still rubbed some guys the wrong way. For example, some of them were getting upset because on maneuvers, all I carried was my M16 and binoculars, and sometimes a radio. They were toting the mortar itself, the base plate, and the ammo. Ten-pound shells add up in a hurry.

Once I forgot and left my radio in a truck. As punishment, one of the lance corporals made me do sit-ups in the shower with the water full blast. Then he made me do a plank. That is when you must lie perfectly still, with your body as rigid as a board. Try that sometime for five minutes.

Around this time, I finally found an apartment I liked, a 1,200-square-foot, one-bedroom unit in Oceanside. It was in an apartment complex that was not in the best section of town, but it wasn't a ghetto. We didn't care. We were young newlyweds, and we were happy that the little apartment was ours. And it was awesome that Darlene and I were finally living under one roof as man and wife.

I know this is a period where a lot of young married couples start planning for their futures. I wasn't like that. By this time, I had two years as a Marine, and all I really thought about was my career in the Corps. That's probably because the scuttlebutt at the base was picking up. There were rumors of a Marine Expeditionary Unit (MEU), where Marines are on ships, heading for a deployment on foreign soil. In our case, that would likely be Iraq or Afghanistan. We were all aware of the growing insurgencies in both countries, although Iraq was the priority of the U.S. military then. So a deployment to Iraq was a distinct possibility. And that meant combat.

But first I would undergo one last round of training at the Marine Corps Mountain Warfare Training Center in Bridgeport, California. Created to train Marines for the Korean War, the center is smack in the middle of the spectacular Sierra Madre Mountains. The elevations there reach more than 11,000 feet. In winter, you are looking at tons of snow and temperatures that reach 20 degrees below zero.

Fortunately, we were doing the summer package. But before we shipped out of Bridgeport, I was told that the base dentist had decided that my wisdom teeth, which came in nice and straight, must come out anyway. All four of them. I decided to have them all yanked the same day. Hey, why prolong the pain? After the operation, the doctor sent me on my way with a script for a couple of days of painkillers. No refills, of course. Naturally, the guys in squad bay rode me like crazy when I walked in. But they shut up fast when I tilted my head back and blood and spit poured out of my mouth. Even the guys who were considered the serious pranksters realized that this was no joke.

And so, a couple of days later, swollen mouth and all, I boarded the bus for the seven-hour drive to Bridgeport, a real treat when every bounce of the bus sends a lightning bolt of pain through your jaw. On arrival, I was immediately assigned to a new company and a new platoon. And of course, the Marines there wanted to harass the new guys. One of their favorite pranks was what they called the "cracker challenge," where you have to eat the two crackers in your MRE kit. They're big and hard. Fortunately, with my swollen mouth, I got a pass.

Whether summer or winter, the Bridgeport program trains you in all ways for mountain warfare. They build up your high-altitude endurance with tons of hikes and maneuvers. You learn how to climb mountains, rappel down mountains, and construct rope bridges over ravines. We learned about altitude sickness and how to treat it. I'm told they now have a program for mountain horsemanship, very handy for Afghanistan, but not when I was there. I did learn how to handle pack mules, though. Even though mine was a summer package, on one of our last hikes it snowed pretty good. Imagine three of us Marines spending the night on the ground with only a flimsy poncho liner (a "woobie," in Marine lingo) to cover us. We shivered like hell. Really made you appreciate that Southern California weather in Pendleton.

After mountain training, we returned to Pendleton and sunny weather, but the base now had a different vibe. Things were heating up, especially in Iraq, where the al-Qaeda attacks were escalating. We began doing workups for being deployed on a ship. They put us in amphibious vehicles, six or eight guys packed in like sardines with all our gear. Then we blasted through the waves and went out farther in the ocean, to the big Navy troop transports.

There we learned the finer points of how to live on a ship; it's no pleasure cruise, believe me. There are some thirty or forty guys in one small berthing area, with only two toilets. We slept in triple-decker bunks. My nose was about three inches from the rack above me. But being packed in like a sardine is an exciting part of being a Marine; you're at sea and headed somewhere, hopefully to fight. The one thing about being a Marine is the discipline you learn and the confidence that comes from tackling some of the worst possible scenarios anyone could imagine.

After all the training, my time to deploy was finally here. I said my good-byes to my wife. Now I was officially part of a Marine Expeditionary Force. We were put out to sea in the transport, on the way to Guam and Singapore.

Or so I thought.

SEVEN

IN COUNTRY: THE FIRST BLAST

WHEN I SAID GOODBYE TO DARLENE IN SAN DIEGO, IT WASN'T EX-actly an intimate parting. How could it be with her parents there, too? They were hovering around us like drones. I had no idea where I was going beyond Guam and Singapore, just that I was on a deployment. I remember, though, that my wife thought it was odd that I showed very little emotion. For me, there were no tears. I guess I was psychologically building a wall between Darlene and me, in the sense that I was thinking more about what lay ahead, not behind. I had some rank now, having met the requirements to become a lance corporal. I remember feeling excited. I guess joy would be too strong a word—maybe keen anticipation is more like it. After all, I'm a Marine. If it's combat ahead, well, that's what I signed up for.

My troop transport was part of a small fleet sailing west in the Pacific. For the life of me, I can't remember all the ships that were with us—whether we had an aircraft carrier, destroyers, or whatever as escorts. Anyway, I can't say I got all that excited about my first overseas cruise. I spent very little time on deck, hanging out in my bunk and using the boat's gym instead. It was next to the engine room and reeked of fumes.

On board, my new unit, Lima Company of Third Battalion, did what we always do—drill, exercise, attend classes, and clean and fire our weapons at targets on the aft decks of the ship. No, I didn't get to fire mortars. The idea of firing these lethal shells into the ocean—killing God knows what kind of marine life—was not even a remote possibility. The Navy doesn't allow it.

Guam was to be our first port of call. Now Guam, as you may know, is a U.S. Territory. It figured prominently in the war in the Pacific during WWII and is quite accustomed to the seeing American servicemen in all their forms. Usually, before we hit a port, we got a lecture on the local customs—what to do and, more important, what not to do. Turned out there is quite a bit of leeway for a footloose Marine on Guam.

I had made several good friends in Bridgeport who were now my shipmates. (For the life of me, I can't remember any of their names now.) Several of us decided we'd rent a car as soon as we landed. So, when we departed the ship, we loaded up our gear and rode into town, a low-slung oceanside village of a few thousand people. The first thing we did was rent a hotel room, one room for all five of us. Next, we did what most young Marines do in a port of call. We went drinking. Boozing it up is routine for most young guys, but in the Marines, it also cements the bonds between brothers. True character can often emerge from the haze of alcohol.

We did manage to avoid the town brothel, called—no kidding—Seven Floors of Whores. The word was that the Shore Patrol was all over the place. Any Marine anywhere near the brothel would be picked up and taken back to the ship.

Now that's not to say we didn't enjoy ourselves. I don't claim to remember everything about that night, but I do recall some highlights. For one, I had the best mojito I ever had. I also recall drinking an Angry Hulk, which is made from Captain Morgan Rum and Mountain Dew. I think we skipped out on the tab for several of those bizarre concoctions. And even though I was a married man, I do seem to remember at some point at one of the clubs we wandered into—not a strip club, but close—I was pulled up on stage by some girl. She made me sit in a chair while she took my shirt off and playfully slapped me with my belt. But, committed young husband that I was, I made sure my pants stayed on.

The next morning, hangovers and all, we decided to visit this touristy spot we heard about from the locals. It had a waterfall and, inside the falls, a tomb where a Japanese soldier, unaware that the war was over, hid out for years before starving to death. The experience was exhilarating! Yet, it was bittersweet in the sense that there we were amid such beauty and, at the same time, realizing the pain and fear that Japanese soldier surely must have felt. That is one of the conundrums of war. While you are trained to eliminate the enemy, they still are human beings, and that realization can at times mess with your head. But, the South Pacific sun, the clean, cascading water, the tiny prisms of light that splashed off your head—this was one hell of a change from a cramped, below-decks berthing area stinking of forty Marines! The folks in charge were cool, and they let us dive off the waterfall to our hearts' content.

We also went snorkeling. Being guys, when we happened upon a sea cucumber, there was great excitement. Sea cucumbers, you may know, emit a viscous white liquid as a defense mechanism. You can imagine what we made of that. Later, we found out that the liquid can blind you. Thank God we left it alone. We also paid a visit to a massage parlor. True blue again, I passed on a "happy ending." All in all, Guam was great. No one got hurt, which was a minor miracle. After our brief adventure, we reboarded our ship and set sail for Singapore.

Somewhere between Guam and Singapore, some 3,000 miles, the word came down. We were bound for Iraq. More troops had been deployed, and the mission was now a counterinsurgency. The level of violence had increased to a virtual civil war. That was all I could think about as we hit Singapore. We had been briefed about how strict the laws were there. For example, you can get arrested for spitting on the sidewalk. For more serious stuff, you can get publicly lashed. I went ashore only once, and not for long. And forget buying souvenirs there. Everything is superexpensive, and as a married man, I couldn't spend a lot of money because of the dispensing system in the military. It works like this: my wife and I had a joint checking account, and if I did choose to take out, let's say, $500 for gifts or whatever, all she would see is that $500 was missing from my paycheck. That could be a marital disaster. So, I was a good guy and spent next to nothing.

The trip by sea was almost 4,500 nautical miles from Singapore to Kuwait. The plan was for us to disembark in Kuwait. We sailed through the Indian Ocean and up the Persian Gulf. On board, things were quieter now, more introspective. We started getting classes in basic Arabic. Maybe the idea of combat was playing on some of our nerves, mine included. For example, back in Bridgeport, I was assigned to a Fire Indirect Support Team (FIST). There were four of us: me as the forward mortar observer, a forward artillery observer, a second lieutenant who was the team leader, and a radio operator. This radio operator was a short guy, maybe 5'6", and he had a serious Napoleon complex.

One day, we're firing our M16s at targets on the stern. I'd been taught by several senior lance corporals to have my extra ammo clips pointing backward on my right hip. That way, you can keep your trigger finger on the trigger, while reaching to your right hip, grabbing the new clip butt first, and popping it right in. This saves time, which really comes in handy when someone is shooting at you.

Well, this radio operator, a corporal named Cheshire, approached me one day during target practice. "Peck," he yelled. "Turn your magazines forward." I tried explaining to him that several senior lance corporals had instructed me that my method was the most efficient for reloading. But he wouldn't listen. We argued, but I refused to follow his order. Remember, I'm a lance corporal, so he outranks me.

So, he ratted me out to two senior lance corporals. I know these guys, and I explained myself to them and why I did what I did. They listened and then huddled for a bit. The verdict? "Yeah, Peck, you were right, the magazines should be secured with bullets pointed behind you. But it's the way you argued with him that got me pissed," one of them told me. This lance corporal, a superfit black guy named Rodgers, told me that there had to be "repercussions," and he wasn't kidding. The senior lance corporals hazed me for a half-hour and at one point made me lie down and put my sternum directly on my Kevlar. Sweet Jesus that hurt! But I toughed it out and was proud when Rodgers commented on how strong I was. The thought did occur to me that, maybe subconsciously, my bad-boy behavior at times was triggered by my anger as a kid. I could have done it differently and should have listened to him for the time being and just gone and told someone with a little bit more pull. But being a Marine was helping me smooth that out, and my Marine buddies gave me a new perspective on what it means to be a family. I belonged, but even more importantly, I had *earned* it.

Once we arrived in Kuwait, we disembarked and reported to this huge staging camp. It was weird. The place had an imposing maze of concrete barriers, a foot thick and twelve feet high. You could not go off-base, so there was no interaction with Kuwaitis whatsoever. They immediately broke my platoon down into sections A and B. Each section consisted of a lead seven-ton truck with upgraded armor (referred to as up-armored), followed by three up-armored Humvees. I was assigned to a Humvee in Section B. With me were a machine gunner (Humvees carry the M240), a staff sergeant who was the commander, and—shit—my "buddy" the radio operator.

Talk about disappointment. Also, we were told right off that we would not be firing our mortars in Iraq. The brass was concerned about collateral damage, that is, accidentally killing or wounding innocent Iraqis as we fired at the real enemies. Also, there was the whole "hearts and minds" thing. So, basically, I was told I was going to be the driver.

A driver? That wasn't what I signed up for, and it really pissed me off; I wanted to fight, to blast the enemy with mortar shells or unleash my M16 in a real firefight. Maybe out of frustration and maybe out of boredom, I went to the base PX the night before we were supposed to drive to Iraq and bought a whole case of Starbucks Frappuccinos. I stayed up all night in the Humvee, drinking all the Frappuccinos and playing video games on my little handheld phone. When it came time to mount up the next morning, I was so tired I could barely see, and I had a very long drive ahead to Iraq. Well, for once I got lucky. The Humvee wouldn't start! So, we hopped a ride in a troop carrier and immediately went to sleep for at least six hours.

When I woke up, I was in Iraq.

At first, we rolled into a Central Operating Base (COB), near Baghdad. The COB is where Marines first arrive in the country before getting their assignments and where they do their R&R when they have a break. The base was huge. It had a chow hall, a PX, showers, and even a McDonald's and a Kentucky Fried Chicken. But I wasn't there long. My destination was the infamous Al Anbar province in western Iraq, where I would spend the next three months on patrol.

Al Anbar, as I would learn, has some flat grassland around the Euphrates River, but it is mostly desert. Temperatures during the day can exceed one hundred ten degrees. Out there in the desert, where we were, conditions are primitive. At night, we would circle up the vehicles and sleep inside them. Or sometimes we would sleep on the roof of the Humvee if there was a nice breeze and we judged the area relatively safe. And if we got lucky, we would find a shady place where we could sleep outside.

During the day, we did mounted patrols, driving around in Humvees. We'd introduce ourselves to the Iraqis and tell them we were there to help. I felt bad about what was happening to their country and sympathized a bit with their suspicion of Americans. I mean, terrorists were their real enemy, but now they had to deal with heavily armed—and I'm sure scary—Marines. And of course, we were always trying to spot the enemy, to engage. But we were wary of everyone. The Iraqi who smiled at you today might be the one shooting at you tomorrow.

The rules of engagement were clear in Iraq. If we saw someone dig-ging—presumably to plant an IED—we could shoot them on the spot. If we saw someone with a weapon, again we could shoot them on the spot. No questions asked. Now, I never saw anyone do that, but we could. (The rules changed in Afghanistan. There, you actually had to see someone putting the IED in the ground before shooting. Different presidents, I guess.)

Out in the desert, our hygiene was awful. There were no showers out there, of course, and we got really nasty. Basically, we stunk. At one point, I could take off my trousers and they would stand on their own. My hair had grown out, and it got so oily and dirty I could actually spike it up. When we did get back to the COB, even showers weren't enough. I would need baby wipes to really get clean.

As for the Iraqis, we encountered them on patrols, sometimes in vil-lages, sometimes in random collections of huts. There was an Iraqi market we frequented where they sold ice, Iraqi food, Cokes, candy, and stuff like that. These folks were pretty friendly. I remember one guy offered me an Iraqi cucumber. To someone who hadn't had fresh food in forever, it was incredibly delicious. We also learned to love their fruit drinks, which actu-ally had chunks of fresh fruit. The first time I had a mango drink, I felt this chunk of something in my mouth and spit it out. But it was just mango. We went through tons of these fruit drinks.

There was also a Marine truck that came by every so often with stuff like candy bars, sodas—I even bought a Microsoft Zune.

Above all, we always had to be on guard. You never knew who to trust. Like I said, that friendly Iraqi might soon have you in his gun sights. Even the kids could be a problem. For example, we secured water tanks and MRE containers on the back of our Humvees. The kids would try to steal them. And they would throw rocks at us and worse. I remember this one kid who aimed a slingshot at me. He fired a rock so hard it cracked the fiberglass on my gun mount. Imagine if that rock had hit me! (I had my revenge on him later. At one point, we rode around tossing soccer balls to the kids—Hearts and Minds stuff. Well, I spotted this kid. I took out a ball, and making sure he saw it, I stabbed the ball with my knife, making it useless. Then I tossed it to him.)

In those first early days, we used our trucks as guard posts. It was very hard to stay awake. At one point, I took to stuffing instant Folgers coffee between my lips and gums, just like dipping snuff, and mostly that worked. But there was one time I fell asleep, if only for a few minutes. Unlucky for me, a corporal spotted me and "turtle-fucked" me. That's where one guy slams his Kevlar into yours. Believe me, I woke up in a hurry.

After a couple of months, though, we got our own forward operating base. Combat engineers came in and erected hescos. These are big walls made of chain-link wire, with big burlap bags mounted on them. The burlap bags are then filled with sand. They make for very good cover and fence us in. At first, there was nothing inside the walls, just us Marines. But eventually we got big tents—big enough for about twenty guys to sleep and walk around in—plywood floors to walk on, cots, showers, and even hot chow, a real treat after eating MREs for weeks on end. When we weren't on patrol, it was boring. We passed the time working out, playing video games, and bullshitting, with the occasional call home on a satellite phone.

Before long, we also got an "eye in the sky" tower—an optical device that allowed us to scan the countryside, kind of a land-based, very high-tech periscope. It was equipped with night-vision capabilities and had to be manned 24/7. As an FOB, we now had the enemy's full attention. A few times they lobbed mortars into our compound, using 60mm hand-held tubes fired off the back of pickup trucks. Then they would haul ass. I don't recall anyone getting killed by mortars, but there was one guy a shell landed close to who developed nervous tics. After an attack, we would pile into vehicles and try to find them, but we never did.

Meanwhile, the war was closing in more on us. In early 2007, the Coalition troops had launched what was known as "the surge," committing more troops to drive al-Qaeda out of Iraq. But al-Qaeda fought back hard. I remember this one really cool guy, Steve Stacey. He wasn't in my platoon, but he and some guys came into our FOB for a little R&R. They had their own FOB, but it wasn't much—just an abandoned house that they had built up with sandbags. One day we got a call. Along with our lieutenant and SSGT Robinson and my buddy Werbleck, I drove the Humvee over to that house. Turns out that Stacey had been laying prone on the top of that house, standing guard, when he was shot and killed. The sniper had put a bullet right through his throat, between his Kevlar and the neck protector that is part of our flak jackets. It was a helluva shot.

We came to learn that the sniper who did it was somewhat famous in our sector, I guess like the Iraqi sniper in *American Sniper*. (I don't go to war movies. Hey, I've lived it!) In fact, he shot another Marine in the throat on top of that same building, but unlike Stacey, this guy lived. I heard later that we eventually got the sniper, but I can't remember the details. Honestly, we didn't know a helluva lot about any of our enemies, whether they were Al Qaeda, Taliban, or whatever. We only knew they were trying to kill us any way they could. But maybe it made us more determined to complete the mission and do what we were trained to do.

Looking back, I do remember a few vehicles getting blown up by IEDs, but I don't recall anyone getting killed as a result. But around this time, our SSGT. Robinson started having heart problems and got sent back. A CPL Bowman replaced him, but now we were down to three vehicles on patrol. I was in the first vehicle, sitting on the back of a seven-ton up-armored truck. It wasn't great. When we stop, I have to look closely at the ground, then jump down about six feet—with gear on. Obviously, there's always the chance that would I land on an IED. Or sprain my ankles. I hated it, so I started nagging Werbleck about becoming the machine gunner.

It's odd, especially since we would spend a lot of time together and even get wounded at the same time, but I have only vague recollections of Werbleck. All I remember is that he liked to wear baseball caps with the bill unfolded. But we did get along really well. In fact, he finally agreed to let me man the machine gun.

He showed me the "diss and ass," that is, how to dissemble and assemble the M240, a belt-fed weapon that can spew out over 600 rounds a minute. I got so good I could do it in a minute and a half. So now when we patrolled, I was the machine gunner in the lead vehicle and Werbleck was the driver. (Sad to admit, it's around this time when I picked up a nasty cigarette habit.)

I recall one patrol where I was left alone in the seven-ton. The other three vehicles had bugged out, and I apparently did not get the word. Suddenly, this Marine came running up. "What the hell are you doing?" he yelled at me. He jumped behind the wheel, and we drove about 400 meters to where all the others were. They were all firing on this house. They started screaming at me, "Get the gun up! Get the gun up!"

At first, I couldn't get the damn 240 to fire. Thankfully, on the third try, the gun worked. So, I joined in, raking the house with rapid fire. Somebody called, "Cease fire." We never even went in to investigate the house. We just left. Things like that happened on a regular basis. Another time, for example, Werbleck was in the 240 turret when a sniper bullet hit the side of our Humvee. We never found out where the shot came from.

We did wise up enough to fashion a kind of box made of that hesco material around the seven-ton. Now you couldn't see the gunner if you were behind the truck or to the side of it. We called it a "sniper hide."

There's also a feature on our Humvees called a HALO system. If a vehicle catches fire, the HALO is designed to put it out. One day, I accidentally hit the HALO switch. There was this blast that sounded like fireworks, and the whole side of the truck was covered in this white stuff. Well, Rodgers—remember, Rodgers is this superbuilt, supertough Marine who hazed me on the ship—panics and bolts from the vehicle. He's running around screaming that we hit an IED. As you can imagine, Rodgers was the butt of jokes for weeks.

But around August, something happened that wasn't funny at all. We had been pushing our patrols outside of our official Area of Operations (AO). We weren't doing any cowboy stuff, taking excessive risks or anything, and I don't recall being especially apprehensive about it. In fact, it was a welcome break from some of our heavily traveled patrol routes; remember, we were eager to get into some shooting situations.

About two kilometers out from our base was this road that was the only way in or out of a village where we suspected the pickups with mortars hid after firing at us. We headed west, past the village I had earlier machine-gunned. At first, we drove over barren fields—the ride was incredibly bumpy—but soon we discovered another road that led right back to our base.

On this road, we found a smaller road that led to a small hut. We drove up, and I stayed on the 240 while the guys went in to investigate. What they found was a big mound of ammonium nitrate under a tarp. Ammonium nitrate is used to make fertilizer, but it can also make bombs and IEDs. (Indeed, we had an ongoing program where Iraqi farmers could exchange ammonium nitrate fertilizer for fertilizer without the nitrate.) A cache this big was clearly trouble.

We called in for an Explosive Ordnance Disposal (EOD) team, which took forever to arrive. It was night by the time they got there. They had to inspect the mound, inform everyone that they were going to blow it up (otherwise people might freak), and, finally, blast it into oblivion. Then they left. We closed out our security and left, too. I was sitting in the little sling right below the 240. It's night, so we all had on night-vision goggles, which restrict your vision. There's not much light out, so it's tough to pick out anything on the ground, even with goggles.

That's when the shit hit the fan. We rolled right over a pressure plate IED. The blast launched me upward, smashing my head into the butt of the 240. I was still conscious but couldn't think straight. Instead of crawling out of the truck through the doors, I crawled all the way over the gun, fell on the hood, and leaped to the ground. I stumbled around. They told me later all I did was scream, "Where is my Microsoft Zune?" Werbleck cracked his head on the steering wheel, and our commander hit his head on a window.

A corpsman pulled the three of us behind the truck and asked us questions. I couldn't answer any of them. All I cared about was the Zune. They rushed us back to our base, and the head corpsman again asked us all these questions. I could not even remember my name.

The next thing I knew, I was lying on a stretcher in a helicopter, Werbleck beside me, on our way to the U.S. airbase in Al Asad, Iraq.

EIGHT

I DON'T KNOW WHY I LOVE YOU

T LEAST I THINK IT WAS AL ASAD. I CAN'T REMEMBER FOR SURE, BUT during Operation Iraqi Freedom, Al Asad, which is near Ramadi, was the second largest military base in Iraq and the place where a lot of wounded Marines were taken. When we arrived, the nurses and medical team separated me, Werbleck, and vehicle commander Thompson from one another. All I can remember from that time is that the doctors kept asking me who I was in a series of questions like "Are you Lance Corporal Peck? Are you John Peck? Are you John Michael Peck?" My response was the always the same: "Nope, nope, nope." Clearly, something was wrong.

I remember lying on a cold examination table with the doctor and nurse trying to make me memorize five words and repeat each one back to them. That is one of the ways they determine not only if I suffered a brain injury, but how severe it was. They asked me to repeat the words *bubble*, *carpet*, and *apple*, but I couldn't recall any of them. Not one word. (It's crazy that I remember those exact words now, but again, that's the TBI for you. Always the gaps.) Anyway, it was obvious to the doctors from this neurological test alone that I had severe memory loss. They quickly determined I had either a concussion or a traumatic brain injury (TBI). Same diagnosis with Werbleck. Thompson, meanwhile, suffered only a concussion and, I learned later, would be sent back to Iraq in just two weeks. No such luck for me.

Werbleck and I were transferred into a medical ward for patients suffering from severe head injuries. I guess I was way too sensitive to light at that point, because all I remember were these harsh fluorescent lights. They were so bright that I began having excruciating migraines. To combat the headaches, the doctors gave me high doses of morphine. For anyone who has ever been on that drug, it's a whopper. Your lights are on, but nobody's home.

Once I was stabilized and had a preliminary diagnosis, and after a few days in the hospital, they decided to fly us to Landstuhl, Germany, a town of some 9,000 folks and host to the largest U.S. military hospital outside the United States. (It was founded in 1953, and by 1997 it became the U.S. military's only medical center in Europe that treats wounded guys like me. And I was so heartened to learn later that Landstuhl also has a large organ donation program. Nearly half of the military members who died there donated their organs.) Werbleck and I were put on stretchers and loaded onto a C130. I remember looking over at this one poor guy who had lost what appeared to be both his legs and thinking, *Boy, I wouldn't want to be that guy*. Little did I know.

Landstuhl was surprisingly relaxed for a military installation. While I was being treated there, I could leave the hospital with special passes. I remember this one time Werbleck and I visited a local bar. That was cool. I also remember really liking the nurses, because they told us we could have ice cream any time we wanted. It's those trivial things that count when you've been through a blast.

But despite the good parts of being in Landstuhl, the medical tests were awful, at least for me. I was undergoing the Military Acute Concussion Evaluation (MACE), a standard battery of tests for your memory (short- and long-term), eyesight, speech, balance, motor skills, and cognition. I did very badly. In fact, for some of the longer tests where I had to take on a computer, not only did I perform poorly, but I could barely stay awake.

It turns out I also had severe balance and speech issues in addition to my memory problems. I had a hard time walking in a straight line, standing at attention, doing an about-face, or even being able to aim my weapon properly. My speech was spotty. I occasionally slurred my words and stammered. It was like my brain was giving me commands that I couldn't obey. And to top it off, when the doctors decided I needed an MRI, the scan came back revealing a tear in one of the frontal lobes in my brain. All of this took place in only about a week in Germany. I must say the military medical team was on top of things, as they always are. But traumatic brain injuries can be tricky. Depending upon what external forces hit someone's head, and their severity, what part of the brain was affected, as well as injuries to the scalp and skull, a long-term prognosis is hard to predict. Some patients recover their cognitive, social, and behavioral abilities quickly, while others may never fully recover or die. In my case, my memory was shot.

After all the many tests were done, I got some devastating news. The doctors told me that I could not go back to my unit. No surprise there. The doctors said that my questionable ability to perform my job could, under battle conditions, pose a risk to my fellow Marines. The bottom line: I had no memory and therefore, how could I perform my job? They said I was "deemed a danger to myself and others." And the worst part for me was that I would have to be flown back to the States for more testing. I was crushed. After all my training and years of learning how to be a Marine, now I was a danger to myself and others? Seriously? It was so devastating because all I have ever dreamed about was being a kick-ass Marine. Now, I don't even know how to break down my weapon or remember my commander's name.

They reviewed my service record and decided to call Darlene to let her know about my injury in detail. Darlene then called my mom to give her the bad news. The Casualty Notification Officer—the military personnel specially trained to deal with families when a service member is injured—told them I was injured, but not too seriously. Little did they know at the time that there were other problems that some of my early tests didn't uncover.

Some of those emerged quickly. Like the first time I spoke to my mom on the phone. I called her three days after I was blown up. I remembered her and knew she was my mother but really didn't recognize her voice; I was just talking to her because the doctors told me to. But she did ask me a few questions, and I was able to remember some things here and there. Same with Darlene, although that call was even weirder. Here's how our conversation went down: "Hi, John. Do you know who I am? I'm your wife," Darlene said. I replied, "Who did you say you were again? I don't remember you, and I don't even have a wife."

While Darlene and I had a short but friendly conversation, it left her totally freaked. Soon Darlene began sending me photos of the two of us together to help me remember our marriage, but it didn't jar any memories at all. I still had no idea who she was. I don't recall being angry or frustrated or anything like that. I just remember feeling kind of empty, and more guarded than anything else. But even though I didn't have any emotional connection to Darlene, I still felt terrible that this nice girl was in pain because of me.

All in all, I was in Landstuhl for about two and a half weeks. While I had very few memories of my life before the blast, it didn't stop me from having a little fun with Werbleck, who, luckily, I did remember. I'm sure at that point my impulse control might have been a bit off. That became obvious when I ventured off-base once with this Army chick that Werbleck and I chatted up. She and I decided to get tattooed—I got a tribal tattoo on one arm, a Maori kind of thing. I don't remember what she had done. Later that evening, Werbleck joined us for some local food and beer. We especially loved that Hefeweizen wheat beer! Despite my injury, Landstuhl was a nice break for me. And to add to it, the doctors said I was stable enough to return home.

So, with my new tattoo and my messed-up brain, I was on my way back to the States and Camp Pendleton. They put Werbleck and me on a flight, and our families were told exactly when we would arrive. Once we landed in San Diego, though, it was funny. Protocol demanded that Werbleck and I be put on gurneys and taken by ambulance to the Naval Medical Center, better known as Balboa Hospital.

My mom couldn't make it since she was in Illinois, but Darlene was waiting there for me when we arrived. The moment she saw me, she had this big smile on her face. I just stuck out my tongue. I have no clue why. Not my finest moment.

Werbleck and I were at the hospital for several hours, as they thoroughly checked us out. After they felt we were okay to be released, we were discharged. They also gave us the phone number of the contact person who would be responsible for arranging all our future medical appointments. I said goodbye to Werbleck as he left the hospital with his family.

Now it was just me and Darlene. Even though she was a very nice person, to me she was a complete stranger. The problem was, she was also my wife.

So, with me not knowing who Darlene was, and Darlene freaked out that I didn't remember her, we returned to our small apartment in Oceanside for what would become among the strangest times in my life. I was married to a woman I didn't know, and she was married to a man she loved but couldn't get through to.

I was surprised that Darlene was so patient with me and that she didn't seem to be particularly upset, at least in the beginning. In fact, Darlene acted more like my occupational therapist during those first few weeks we were back home. It was obvious that she really loved me and was totally committed to helping me remember our married life together. I appreciated her dedication, but, to be honest, I didn't have any feelings for her. Except that she seemed like a nice person. She came up with a plan, and together, we set about the task of recovering my memory of her and— for that matter— myself. Hell, I couldn't even remember any of my Marine stuff. That was the worst part of it for me. The Marines were my life, and now I no longer had any idea what a pugil stick was or even a mortar.

Darlene was a truly sweet girl. And I was impressed with her researching what she should do to help me get back to where I was before the blast. She would try to help me regain my memory by asking me personal questions like "Do you remember our wedding?" or "What was your job in the Marines?" Looking back, even though I couldn't remember why I loved her, her patience was something that stuck with me.

When my mom would come to visit us, or when we spoke by phone, she would do the same thing. My mom would constantly ask me stuff like "John, do you remember when you were a child you took me out for my birthday?" Or "John, do you remember the house we lived in Rockford?" But, unfortunately, all I could remember was bits and pieces of my life before the blast. It was devastating! There were nights I would lie in bed trying to recall the most basic memories. It was like my brain was stuck in neutral. Sometimes I was so frustrated that I thought I would never be the same person I was before. And I felt bad that I couldn't rekindle my feelings for Darlene. But, like the determined Marine I was, I decided to forget the pity party and turn my full attention and time to making a go of our marriage.

It must have been hell for Darlene, too. For one thing, I wasn't allowed to drive. So, almost every day she had to take off work—at the time she worked in a Gap store—and drive me to my appointments at Balboa, a forty-five-minute trip each way. And it wasn't as if I was making progress at the hospital. In those MACE memory tests, I could only remember the last few words of any sequence of words.

After a few months of Darlene taking me to my therapy sessions and doctor appointments, I was still having a tough time. While I could give her a hug, and even hold her hand, I still couldn't find the reasons why I loved her. I really couldn't remember anything like that at all. I felt awful that nothing I tried to reconnect with her was working. Nothing at all.

But I have to give Darlene credit for sticking with me, and I know that wasn't easy. I do remember one happy time we had together when she surprised me with an Xbox 360. I even said to her, "Oh my God, Darlene, thank you, I love you so much." They may have been hollow words, I'm sad to say. But as soon as I set the Xbox up, I spent most of the night in my pajamas playing video games. I'm sure that wasn't the response she had hoped for. But the truth was that my personality was changing, and I wasn't the same guy she married, or I had even remembered. Before the blast, I was talkative, tenacious, and involved in everything. There was no challenge I wouldn't take on—no task that was too complicated to complete. After the blast, I became sullen and withdrawn. I wasn't interacting with Darlene—or anyone else, for that matter—and I retreated physically and emotionally. Video games became my best friend. My wife, someone I didn't even recognize, let alone have any feelings for, was still a stranger to me. It was during that period of time when my marriage really began to unravel.

One morning, I woke up and decided I had to be straight with Darlene. I did my normal routine of going to my appointments, and then I decided that I finally had to tell Darlene just how I felt. It was a heart-wrenching conversation, but it had to be done. "Darlene," I said, "I can't do this anymore. I'm sorry, but I'm not finding the spark. And I seriously don't remember why I love you." She was taken aback. "Is this a joke, John?"

"No, Darlene, I'm sorry," I said, "but I don't remember you, and, as much as I've been trying, there's nothing there." She turned her head away and burst out crying. When she got herself together, she said, "John, we can get help, we can work on this." I had to be honest with her, though it was heartbreaking for me. I told her as gently as I could, "Darlene, you don't understand, and it's not your fault, but there's a part of me that, no matter how I try, doesn't love you."

That, as you can imagine, was the beginning of the end of our marriage.

Darlene and I were still living together as husband and wife in Oceanside, but it was increasingly uncomfortable living with a woman who was basically a stranger. To wake up in the morning not knowing why I was there, or my wife wanting to be intimate with me and my wanting nothing to do with her. It was like I was living in someone else's shoes. In addition, my career as a Marine was by no means certain.

At the time, I wasn't reporting to the base. Instead, I had all these medical appointments at the Balboa Navy Hospital in San Diego. The doctors and therapists were working with me to regain what I had lost in terms of my memory and to help me with some balance and speech issues. Military doctors, by necessity, have considerable expertise in this area. In fact, at Walter Reed, they have a state-of-the-art facility dedicated to helping warriors with TBIs heal both physically and psychologically.

At the time, Darlene and I had two cars, one that her dad had given her and the other was hers. I was carless. While we still tried to work on things, it wasn't too long after that I decided to move out and return to a small squad bay on base. In fact, Darlene recently reminded me that on a Sunday I told her that I loved her, and then while she was at work on Monday, I packed up my things and left, never warning her that I was moving out. That's what a traumatic brain injury does, folks. It makes you do and say things you might have never done or said if you were "normal." Like I said earlier, the TBI leaves you with gaps, in this case a major hole where empathy should be, especially toward someone you loved.

Friends who had wondered what was going on with me and Darlene could see I wasn't the same person that I was before my injury. Like I said earlier, before, I was much more outgoing, and I always was up for going out and doing things. Postblast, I became more of a shut-in. I never wanted to leave the house or even interact with my buddies, friends, or family. This was my new reality. In fact, one of my friends brought this to my attention when he said, "Dude, you used to go out and do things, and now you're not doing anything but sitting around playing video games." He was right. The one thing people should know if they have to deal with someone who has a traumatic brain injury is that no two are alike. Everyone's brain injury affects them in separate ways. Some guys I knew couldn't control their anger, a side effect that may explain why doctors initially worried I could be a danger to myself and others. Some guys couldn't even count to ten, and there was one wounded warrior who forgot how and when to eat or the need to take a shower. Your brain is your everything—your mission control center—and mine was far from what it was before the blast. Before the blast, I was on top of my game. I could calculate and evaluate complex data, implement plans, and take care of both my military life and home life. Now I was hesitant, unsure. I couldn't understand how to balance my checkbook, drive my car, or do simple tasks like making a shopping list. Often, I would simply draw a blank.

It was also weird being back on base alone in my room; I had to get used to it again. I knew I was still a Marine, but for the life of me, I couldn't remember what that title meant. What the heck? But no matter what, every day I would go to therapy and they would help me begin to get my memory back. First, it was simple things like repeating numbers, then seeing if I could say them backwards. There would be other sessions to help me regain my balance. I would walk up and down the hallway more times than I can count to keep me steady. During that time, I was determined to overcome my disability and be the same guy I was before I was injured. I knew it would be among the toughest times in my life, but heck, I'd been through much worse before. I wasn't about to quit. And it really helped that I made a visit back to Illinois and spent a week with my mom. We sat around talking for hours, looking through old scrapbooks—anything to jog my memory. I remember telling my mom about a dream I had that on my next deployment, I wasn't going to return home the same. That I would die or be critically injured. How weird was that?

Luckily, over a short amount of time, my memory began to improve. Soon I was able to recite simple numbers. I could also do more complex tasks like adding more numbers to a sequence and stuff like that. There was so much I had to relearn. I'm not going to lie. This was a terrible time in my life; very disturbing. When you were used to being able to perform complex tasks, and doing them very well, I might add, not even being able to even count from one to ten—well, that stinks. In fact, there were many times I was so frustrated that I wanted to give up. But I was a Marine, and the one thing about that is that giving up is not an option. Hey, if I could get through boot camp and all my specialized training, surely I could relearn enough to get back to where I was before the blast. Finally, that iron will to survive—maybe even to thrive—was beginning to stir.

Among the most important things I had to learn was how to drive again. I had to go to therapy first to make sure I could understand the driver's test and, of course, operate a vehicle. That would have been a no-brainer for me before my injury—remember, I'm a guy who could whip around a seven-ton, up-armored truck—but it was tough getting behind the wheel again and knowing what to do. Still, I persevered and finally passed my driver's exam. But the truth is, while I had a basic understanding of simple tasks, it was very difficult to relearn how to drive and how to do things I did with ease before—like cooking. I was really missing that part of me.

Despite months of testing and therapy and progress, I still had only bits and pieces of my memory; none was of Darlene. That did make me sad at times—not because I had feelings for her, but because I had put her through all this pain. And the weirdest thing about my recollections was that most of the memories that did come back were bad; some were about my childhood—especially being rejected by Mike and abused by Adam. But there were a few happy memories, too, like the Sunday afternoon trips I took with my mom, our shopping trips together, and how she stood up for me when I didn't want to play the cello. These memories were comforting. They signaled there were better times ahead if I could push through.

And I was making progress, however slowly. I figured that I was injured in August 2007 and was back in the States before my birthday in September. But I still wasn't in good enough shape to be with my unit for our second deployment, this one to Okinawa in mid-2008.

I have a theory that you should never look back at anything you did in life and wish you could change it. The past is the past, and, besides, I had too much bad stuff to deal with. One thing I did know: I wasn't ready to quit being a Marine.

NINE

FINALLY, A MARINE AGAIN

M Y UNIT, THE GOOD OLD 3/1, RETURNED FROM IRAQ IN LATE 2007. I learned that they had first sailed from Kuwait to Australia. Best of all, on the way home there was a layover in Hawaii. Families were encouraged to fly out to meet their Marine and see how a leatherneck lives on board a ship. In fact, one family member per Marine could sail back from Hawaii to California with them. I would have loved that, because without the blast it would have been Darlene.

But the truth was, at that time in my recovery, I wasn't terribly sorry I missed that mission. After all, you will recall I'm not much of a romantic about travel on the high seas. And besides, at the time I didn't really know who I was, what I was doing, or why I was doing it. Heck, I didn't even recognize my old buddies like Gilbert or Kelly when my unit got back.

One of the few things I do remember clearly is hearing that another one of my pals, Martin Kelly, the goofball himself, was on report for an unauthorized absence when he failed to show up for morning formations for about a week. It didn't really register with me until I returned home one day and found him sitting in my Oceanside apartment by himself; Darlene was at work. But even then, I didn't fully recognize one of my best Marine buddies. (Sadly, his "Boot shrug," that "Hey, I'm a stupid boot" routine, didn't cut it this time. They busted him from lance corporal, reduced him to half-pay, and put him under several other restrictions. Even Martin couldn't be cheery about that.)

In terms of my Marine duties, my only real task was to get better and try to recover some of my memory. I did these Marine Corps Institute courses, which are intended to help you further your Marine career, with books on things like leadership and mathematics. The books have tests, and you are graded on your answers. My grades weren't very good. It was another frustrating time for me because I prided myself on having a good memory and working to complete tasks. And here I was with a brain injury, not even being able to remember the basics, let alone recognize my buddies.

I was assigned to a "boot drop," which you may remember is when they bus over a load of boot camp graduates to the School of Infantry (SOI) at Pendleton—a process I had gone through some three years earlier. But now my job was to walk these new guys around, get them oriented, help them with their new gear, and so on. It's not exactly why I enlisted. Then again, my combat injury was a constant reminder of why I wanted to be a Marine in the first place. Marines, remember, seek combat. Overcoming obstacles, even injuries, is a big part of that.

I was happy that I was still nominally attached to the 3/1, but still on very limited duty. The unit was performing military exercises and going on hikes, but I wasn't allowed to go with them. It's like putting candy in front of a person on a diet. And my medical appointments were getting a lot more spread out, too. In many cases, the doctors were simply waiting to see if my memories would come back. I had a lot of time on my hands, which, for a person with a TBI, was tough. Before, I couldn't wait to learn and complete complicated tasks, and now I was just hanging around hoping my brain would return to normal. But, despite the issues I had, I felt this grim determination to get back to my unit, to be a sharp Marine again. Iraq was winding down, but the war with the Taliban in Afghanistan was heating up. Men would be needed.

Things changed for the better in April. The word came down that the 3/1 would be deployed to Okinawa, a Pacific Island some 1,000 miles southwest of Japan. That was the scene of some of the bloodiest fighting of the Second World War. The Allies suffered around 50,000 casualties, including almost 3,000 dead Marines. Now the island is home to a Marine base where they teach jungle warfare.

Traumatic brain injury or not, I was hell-bent on going with them. I knew my unit would need four forward observers (FO) for its mortar teams. One possible route for me was to become one of those FOs. I somehow managed to be the person they assigned to find the four most experienced guys to complete this mission. But I didn't have much success. The only Marines who had the experience needed were me—the guy who lost his memory—and Cpl. Robinson, who I knew from Iraq. But Robinson wasn't sure if he was going to reenlist. Oddly enough, one of the guys I did train and who was qualified to go was Justin Hill. One of the ironies was that Justin—who helped Darlene and me move into our first apartment—eventually ended up marrying her after we finally were divorced in 2008. I guess the two of them found a spark. I wasn't angry, though. After all, I wanted Darlene to find happiness again, and emotionally, I didn't love her. So, there was no hurt involved for me. I'm not the kind of person who says, "Woe is me." I just keep on going.

But, no matter how hard I pushed, the doctors weren't going to let me go on any missions under any circumstances. I was still rated as unfit for active duty. So, I stayed. Even though I felt like shit, I knew I had to do whatever they told me to. I did understand that my recovery would be slow, but I was growing impatient with things not coming back to me as quickly as I had hoped.

Now I was part of that illustrious group called the "RBU," which means "Remained Behind Unit." This group consists of Marines who are short-timers, others who have gotten into trouble, be it drugs or otherwise, and medically restricted guys. Around this time, I was promoted to corporal, which was huge for me. Despite my TBI, I managed to qualify with the rifle, time in rank, physical condition, and several other factors. So, I was put in charge of the medical group, which consisted of about twenty guys. I was stoked! Finally, I was beginning to get my mojo back. (One of the guys in this group, a lance corporal named Avila, turned out to be the second Marine shot through the neck by that sniper I told you about. The sniper killed Steven Stacey, but Avila survived.)

Part of my responsibilities with these guys was to learn the HIPAA laws. That was the Health Insurance Portability and Accountability Act, which is all about the privacy and security of protecting patients' medical information. The classes I needed for HIPPA were all the way across the base, so clearly, I needed a car. By that time, of course, I no longer had Darlene's old Mercedes. So, I took a trip down to Oceanside, got a car loan, and became the proud owner of a used Dodge Stratus.

I was aware that Marines were fighting and dying in Afghanistan. But I now began one of the dullest seven-month stretches of my Marine career, a period defined by the departure of my unit and their expected return.

Every day, my little group had formation on the grinder. They were a motley crew, to be honest, but at least I was in charge of something again. I had to find out what we were supposed to do that day, then get my guys ready to complete our mission. I went from finding the enemy, sweeping for mines, and killing the enemy to mowing the grass, painting the curbs, and repairing whatever needed repairing. And I had to make sure all my guys were doing what they were supposed to do off the base, like making their medical appointments. I also had to remember to make my own appointments, too. I took my duties seriously, hoping at some point I could go back to active duty and be united with my Marine unit. I can't say I had led an unselfish life to this point, but helping my guys—helping *someone*—I think it struck a chord, a chord that would resonate later.

But, as I said, that was later. Looking back, I was on autopilot for much of this time. Most of my mental energy went to learning more about myself and how to be a Marine again. I did this by watching other Marines, seeing what they regularly did, and listening closely to what they were saying. Reading all those MCI booklets helped, too.

While the memories during my younger years were still hazy, my Marine Corps memories were fresher, so they started coming back sooner. I hate to say it, but in a strange way I now felt free. I wasn't married to a stranger anymore, and I was making progress on being a Marine again. Things were beginning to look up.

By the time 3/1 had returned to the States, it was around the end of the year and I had been through scores of doctor appointments and all kinds of psychological tests. It was time for me to make a life-changing decision. I had been a Marine for more than three years. I had to decide whether to reenlist for another four-year hitch or to get out. I was gung-ho, but the decision wasn't all up to me.

First, I had to get the okay from the doctors. I did several cognitive tests to determine if I was fit for duty. They would ask me questions like "Are you aware of the dangers of being a Marine? Are you aware that you could die on a deployment?" I always answered, "Yes." Soon, the word came back. The doctor said: "Cpl. Peck, you are psychologically okay, but your memory is still bad." And it was. For example, when we were told about an upcoming inspection before my first deployment, I had no trouble remembering the time and the right uniform to wear. Now, I had to write everything down. Word for word. But when push came to shove, the doctors eventually gave me the thumbs-up. I was cleared to get off limited duty. I remember being so excited to finally know, after all my challenging work and pain, that I could go back to finally being a Marine again.

But before I could officially sign my paperwork, I had to run a gauntlet of my superiors. I needed to get approval from all my higher-up guys, the platoon commander, the company commander, the battalion commander, and the battalion sergeant major. I really didn't stand out in any way, but in some cases that was good. About the only thing most of my superiors knew about me was that I got blown up in Iraq. I guess I must have made a positive impression, because they all approved me to serve again.

A guy in the command post put together my reenlistment package and sent it to Marine headquarters. I was told I would remain as a 0341, part of a combat mortar team. I also received a $58,000 reenlistment bonus. (Among other things, the amount of re-up bonuses depends on your rank and, importantly, how much the Corps needed your particular skill at that time.) I told the guy I wanted to go into culinary, and he said this was possible! That was awesome. So, I could do another six months at Pendleton, then one more deployment, and the Marines would send me to the Culinary Institute of America. What an incentive!

As of April 2009, I was a Marine for another four years. I met with a regimental sergeant major, who looked me over and decided I should work in the base gym. So, for the next six months, I folded towels and cleaned exercise equipment. I was basically being paid to sit on my ass and watch people work out. And it was only from 6:00 a.m. until noon—all free time after that. Not a bad gig.

I was also beginning to date again. It didn't feel that strange, given that I had almost no memory of when or why I had married Darlene.

Along with the relaxed schedule, I also caught a break on housing when I put in a request to live off-base. Usually, only sergeants get this, but I told them I had a lot of furniture and really didn't want to pay for storing it. They approved the request in no time, and so despite all the warning signs, I rented a one-room apartment in Temecula, California, a bit north of Pendleton, just in case things with this Myspace chick would work out. Before long, she was living with me, and every so often, her kid would stay over, too. In about a month or two after she moved in, I found myself not just financially supporting her, but her kid, as well. I should have known better. We were all warned early in our military careers that some women would try to hook up with us because we were military men and had steady jobs. This scenario was even more pronounced for officers, and also for wounded warriors like me.

With all this going on, it became clear that I also needed a new car. So, I decided to part with some of my $58,000 reenlistment bonus to buy a black Nissan 350Z. I was quite the dude. With my new car, girlfriend, and apartment, things went well for a while. But before long, I got tired of the drive from Temecula to the base, so the three of us moved to a two-bedroom apartment in Oceanside. Now I had a room for her kid, and the best part was that it was only about twenty minutes to base in my new ride.

But true to form, things began to unravel quickly from there. First, my girlfriend told me she had to visit a friend in North Carolina. Then I somehow found out that she had been sleeping with her drug dealer. She was on my phone plan, and I could see from the list of numbers who she called most frequently. I called the number that came up most often ,and it was her drug dealer. We talked for about ten minutes. Needless to say, it was a very informative and not the most comfortable conversation. And—stupid Marine that I was—I had given her access to my bank account. As soon as I did, I noticed she started taking money out. Big money. I was pissed. So, I told her our relationship wasn't working out and that she and her son should leave. We parted ways, but totaling it all up, I discovered this chick had relieved me of some $15,000. Talk about learning a painful lesson! But the truth was that for me, coming from such a tumultuous background, having ADHD, and now suffering from a traumatic brain injury, I was vulnerable and in need of connection—regardless of who I was connecting with.

Luckily, I still had the apartment, and I got Ian Drewbell, one of the guys from my unit, to move in with me. Drewbell, a soft-spoken, mixed-race kid from Colorado, was a sniper by trade, low-key but deadly. He had also re-upped and received a nice bonus. He too bought a Nissan 350Z, and we became total 350Z nerds. Every weekend, we would work on our cars. We detailed them, and then we started customizing our prize possessions. His became the "Stealth Bomber," since his car was silver. I named mine the "Black Widow." I even added some red paint and cool lights right under the frame. Hey, two Marines driving hot cars—well, you couldn't ask for more of a chick magnet than that. These simple things I did before and now was enjoying again after my recovery made me feel like the Marine—and the man, where women were concerned—that I used to be. It felt great. I realized how my genetically infused personality—that diamond-hard core that helped me cope with disappointment, pain, and abuse—kicked in big-time after my first blast. It allowed me to overcome adversity by compartmentalizing the problem, then closing off the fear to get to the endgame.

I felt good enough to do what I always want to do, have a dog! I got an adorable puppy, in this case a Shiba Inu, a small, agile Japanese breed that resembles a fox. I named him Diesel. When I went to work, I would leave Diesel alone in the kitchen, with a gate to keep him fenced in. Diesel was not the most well-behaved dog in the world, but I loved him despite his numerous transgressions. During the day, he would make a tremendous mess in the kitchen, which you would expect from a young dog. But, just like his old man, he didn't like to be corrected. In fact, he would snap at me when I tried. I think his unruly behavior was karma. What goes around sure comes around, as they say.

But despite my aggravation, the best part was that I knew I would be a full-fledged Marine again. All my sacrifice, all my working to regain my memory, was worth it. The endless therapies—cognitive, emotional, and physical, not to mention having to relearn the basic things I did before such as driving or performing my duties including planning and executing missions as a Marine—were a huge challenge. But I was never the kind of person to give up on anything. I was not about to let a traumatic brain injury get me down or force me to give up on my dream. I had to rally all of my inner strength and fortitude to make it through this crazy time in my life. Just like I had to do when I was a child.

Nor was I about to give up on the fairer sex. Although my first marriage ended in a divorce, and then I got involved with the wrong person, I was always up for trying to find love again. I hung around Pacific Beach a lot, where a lot of the college girls were. Now I wasn't the biggest, baddest Marine around, but I was pretty fit and never had a problem attracting girls.

As luck would have it, I met this cute girl at my apartment complex. Her name was Betty. She was about five foot seven and was from Nashua, New Hampshire. She was married at the time to another Marine. Betty was about my age and had a dog, too, a cute little Yorkie. We got to talking at the dog park one day, and before long we became friends. It was nice to talk to someone who seemed to understand me, and Betty was a good listener.

During those six months when I worked at the gym, Betty and I grew even closer. But sometimes it got weird. Like the time she told me details about her husband, and how their relationship wasn't working out. Sometimes after Betty and her husband argued, she would come over to my apartment. She just wanted to talk. Unfortunately, there were a couple of times when her husband—a tall, lanky dude who I thought was way too big for his britches—would come over and yell at Drewbell and me while we were sitting on our little patio smoking or grilling our dinner. "Why are you guys fucking around with my wife?" he'd yell. "What are you talking about, dude?" we'd yell back. Hell, the truth was that I wasn't even sleeping with her yet. If I wanted to, I could wrap my whole hand around his bicep. I could easily have kicked his ass, but I kept my cool.

One day, Betty told me she didn't want to live with her husband anymore. I was intrigued. I asked her what she wanted to do. Now bear in mind this is a cute girl who wore very form-fitting dresses for her job at a Sprint kiosk in a nearby mall. (For most Marines, that's about all it takes to get their attention.) I told her, "Betty, we really don't have much room here, but I'm sure we can work something out." It was probably a reckless thing to do, but I needed to have a woman in my life. Given my lifelong struggle with abandonment, I think I rushed into my relationship with Betty out of fear of being alone. I wish I had known at the time that this was not the woman I should have attached myself to.

A few nights after Betty moved in, the four of us got drunk—me, Betty, Drewbell, and his girlfriend, who later became his wife. You know how alcohol is often called "liquid courage"? Well, it must have had that effect on Betty, because out of the blue she kissed me; I didn't resist. Betty was becoming more than just a friend. And I really liked her, too. I could see that she had some issues with her current husband. Maybe it was her fault, but I don't know for sure. Remember, I hated the guy and I was infatuated with her. But, maybe because of my TBI, I didn't try to psychoanalyze this person. I was just happy to feel something for a woman again.

After that drunken night, and Betty's kiss, I started to keep away from Pacific Beach and took myself off the dating site. It would be a decision I would come to regret.

TEN

BECOMING A SQUAD LEADER

D URING THOSE SIX MONTHS AT THE GYM, I WAS EITHER WORKING OR working out. And like I said, I had a lot of free time. When I wasn't hanging out with Betty, all my time went to getting stronger, to recovering more of my memories. I continued to do the memory exercises they gave me in the hospital and as part of my outpatient therapy. They would ask me to do things like memorize a story, then repeat key points about the story. Or, repeat a story verbatim. They really didn't help with any advanced type of tasks I could easily do before—that was something I had to relearn on my own. For example, I had to figure out how to work on cars, cook a meal, and all the things I used to do as a Marine. Essentially, any task that didn't come naturally was something I had to figure out; it was a bitch! I would have to work on walking and balance issues, as well. And, of course, Drewbell and I had plenty of time to work on our cars and grill on the patio with Betty. Looking back, injury or no, it was a damn good stretch for this young Marine.

It wouldn't last forever, though. In October, I was reassigned to my old weapons company with Third Battalion, First Marines. They'd received orders for deployment to Afghanistan, so they were pulling people back to begin training for the mission. We were expecting to be sent over in April 2010. The year would prove the deadliest for U.S. troops, with 2,403 KIAs. It would also make Afghanistan our longest war, replacing Vietnam.

I remember chatting with my new company first sergeant. He didn't know me at all. All he knew was that I was blown up in Iraq and had memory problems. He asked me, "How are you doing, corporal?" I told him: "Well, my memory hasn't totally returned, but I've relearned some things and I'm ready and able to readapt to be an active Marine; I'm ready to go."

"Okay," he replied, "You're going back to the 81mm mortar platoon, and in fact, they're right outside." Wow, that was a shock.

I walked out and onto the road, to find the grinder full of cars and high-spirited Marines. It was the day before a three-day holiday weekend, and the Marines always hold a vehicle inspection for guys going off-base. It's a safety procedure, of course, but really just another way they fuck with you. But hey, there they were. My old buddies Ian Gilbert and Martin Kelly, a bunch of guys from my old unit, plus a lot of the guys I walked around at SOI when I first got back from Iraq. Many of them knew me, of course, but I was still having a lot of trouble remembering exactly who they were. Justin Hill was there, too. Him I remembered. Darlene's husband. It was nice to see these guys, but I had to check in with my new platoon sergeant, Gunnery Sergeant Martinez, and my platoon commander, Lt. Saville. I assumed they would tell me I would be a forward observer—that's what I wanted—but here's another quick lesson: never assume anything in the Marine Corps! They told me they already had three FO's (Hill, damn it, was one of them), so there was no need for me. But one of the eight guns that make up a mortar platoon did not have a squad leader. (As you'll recall, each gun has four men—a squad leader, an ammo man, a gunner, and an assistant gunner.)

"Corporal Peck, we're looking at you for squad leader of the eighth gun," they said. It was between me and a corporal named White, who frankly was a bit of a tool. I think they knew that because they said they needed me to prove myself. *How was I supposed to do that?* I wondered.

The answer was the Infantry Mortar Leader Course, a grueling two months of physical training and weapons instruction at the School of Infantry in Pendleton. It's ten hours a day, six days a week, all beginning at 6:00 a.m. Well, I needed it. Remember, I was either driving a truck or Humvee or manning a 240-machine gun during my time in Iraq. I hadn't touched a mortar since my own SOI stint. I wasn't even sure how to assemble the damn thing anymore.

It was all indoor stuff at first, except for the physical training, which I'll get to in a moment. Initially, we sat in a classroom. A Sgt. Blake, a senior guy and a big one to boot, was the instructor. He told us what they would teach over the next eight weeks, and how we would be able to go back and teach the younger guys in our units. I sat in the back of the room. At one point, I yawned really big, no covering my mouth, no muffling the sound, no nothing. Sgt. Blake stopped talking. Looking directly at me, he said, "Peck, the one thing you can do that will piss me off the most is yawn straight up, not covering your mouth. That's one of the worst things you can do."

A great start, huh? You better believe that during the next phase of the program I held my yawns in control, not to mention my mouth. There would be no yawning in the physical training (PT). First, they wanted to see what you can do. I think I managed seventeen or eighteen pull-ups, one hundred sit-ups in two minutes, but my run time sucked. As I said before, I'm a hiker, not a sprinter. But run we did, a good mile from Base Area Fifty-One to Area Fifty-Two, then another half mile or so to the obstacle course, which we did two or three times. Then we ran back to Area Fifty-One.

We're doing this, by the way, in our boots and uniforms, not PT shorts and tees. And there was also the "stick and donut" runs, in which four or five of us run carrying telephone poles or the tires off the seven-ton trucks. And we did all this torture in flak jackets and Kevlars. Afterward, I would shower at the gym and change into a fresh pair of Cammie pants. My sweaty ones went in the back of my car, which began to smell like a gym bag. The PT absolutely whipped my ass into shape.

As for the mortars, they teach you everything about the weapon and all the jobs associated with it. Even though I always thought of myself as a forward observer, I began to really like working in the Fire Direction Center (FDC). They have control over the gun crews when it comes to selecting targets and providing the coordinates, deciding which units will fire, and the type and amount of ammunition that's going to be used for each mission. This really appealed to me. I was always good at math, which came into play heavily here. It was also cool to see the other side of things, what happened when I, as a forward observer, called in coordinates. It tied everything I had learned as a mortar man together and made me feel even more valuable to the Corps.

The FDC is where the squad leader is in combat, and the job is to aim the mortar to hit the target called in by the forward observer. The FDC is the go-between for the forward observers and the gunline. When the FO gets eyes on the target, he or she radios in the coordinates to the FDC. The FDC calculates the information in the Advanced Field Artillery Tactical

Data System, and that data lets everyone know the weather conditions that possibly could affect a round. It's a very technical but necessary function. As I said, I was always good at math, and I got really good at this, too. I was beginning to feel confident that all my hard work to recover from the TBI was finally paying off!

All along, my company first sergeant Balcazaar and Gunny Martinez were getting reports on me. They told me later there were a few times they were worried about me passing. But there was nothing that would stop me now. And it was a hoot for me to see Balcazaar and Martinez at my graduation. I know they were proud of me in their own way, and I was proud of me, too. It was a long road back, but it was worth all the struggles. Hell yeah!

Finally, I was a squad leader.

ELEVEN

BACK IN THE GAME

B Y THIS TIME, I WAS TOTALLY FOCUSED ON THE DEPLOYMENT. I MUST ADMIT that some small part of me was a little worried. This was another combat deployment, and that clearly meant there was a chance of death or another severe injury. I mean, it's just one of those things. I like to think of myself as logical, so just looking at the situation, I had to examine the possibilities realistically. In late 2009, President Obama announced a surge of his own, committing an additional 33,000 troops to Afghanistan. For me, combat was now a distinct possibility. And having just recovered from getting blown up in Iraq, I did not want to go through all that again. Once is more than enough.

But the silver lining was that Betty and I got engaged and were married on Valentine's Day 2010. Unlike my previous marriage, we had a supersmall wedding ceremony with only Betty and I and one of her friends present. We decided to get married in, of all places, Las Vegas. Not in a drive-through Elvis kiosk, but a tiny little church with someone who looked like my grandma presiding. Our honeymoon was only a weekend at the strip, rather than an extended getaway. After all, Betty had been living with me, and I was totally focused on my deployment.

When we got back from Vegas, Betty told me she was a little worried about me leaving, but she was no stranger to the military life. Betty had been around Marines—she was now married to a second Marine, after all—and understood that this was part of the deal. So, she wasn't like,

"Oh, my God, please don't go." The bottom line: this was my job. And I loved it.

Then it got even better. I was assigned my first squad; Lance Corporal Spangler, Lance Corporal Byone, and Private First Class Bulosan.

These guys knew me from my time in the unit before, but they didn't see me as any kind of a leader. None of them had been part of our unit's deployment to Iraq. Spangler and Byone had been to Okinawa, but they had never been in combat. Bulosan had never been deployed, period.

I knew them, but I didn't know how they did their jobs. I had never trained with them, which meant I didn't really know how well trained they were. More important, I didn't know how they were going to perceive me. Would they welcome me? Or would they be thinking, *Hey, who is this guy? He gets injured, he reenlists, and then he disappears for six months. So, they put him in charge? Does he even know how to do his job anymore?* So, naturally, they were wondering if I was going to be a douchebag or a jerk.

So, even though I outranked them as a corporal, and had been deployed, it was still up to me to gain their respect and show them that we could be a good team. That doesn't just happen. You have to create that bond with your guys.

I started working on that during our training. In preparation for Afghanistan, we went to the Marine combat training center in Twenty-Nine Palms, east of Los Angeles in the Mojave Desert, and another base in Yuma, Arizona, for mortar drills and large-scale battalion maneuvers. We were honing our skills at the squad level as a mortar crew, but also in conjunction with larger units, simulating combat conditions. First, the mortars would fire, and then the machine gunners and TOW gunners would open up, softening up the objective for the infantry to come in and clean up. (TOW, by the way, stands for tube-launched, optically tracked wire-guided weapons system. Think of it as a more modern and more lethal version of the World War II bazooka.)

The inspections were nonstop. There were mortar inspections, gear inspections. And then double-checking to make sure everyone packed everything they would need. We had a packing list of stuff to bring, of course, and it was very detailed, like bring three pairs of desert cammies and three pairs of green cammies. If someone in your squad failed an inspection, then we all had to have another one.

After all that, the drills and maneuvers in Twenty-Nine Palms and Yuma, and all the other training and inspections, me and my guys got tighter. They could see that I wasn't a dickhead, that I wasn't going to sit and yell at them for no reason. I'm not trying to say I was the best squad leader, but I wasn't going to make them play stupid games. That's not who I was. I sat down and talked to them a lot, too. And I was straight with them. One of the things I remember talking to them about was how to prepare themselves and their families for the deployment. I said, "Look, you know we're going to Afghanistan. You know there's a chance that someone in our squad of four guys could get injured or one of us could die. You need to prepare your families for this. I'm a prime example. I got injured in Iraq. You need to be ready for that possibility. You need to be mentally strong. Talk to your wife. Talk to your mom and dad, whoever it may be, and tell them, 'This might happen and just be prepared for it.'"

I also tried to tell them about my own experiences on a combat deployment. But I had a tough time because of my traumatic brain injury. I'd try to tell them something, and then at the same time I'd have to pause and think, *Duh, I'm not completely sure I can even remember what Iraq was like*. I could recall bits and pieces of the experience. I could remember where we were and even visualize the market where we got all our fruit drinks. I could see our forward base, but I couldn't remember many of the details.

Overall, though, my short- and long-term memory had improved. It helped that I always wrote stuff down. I always had a notebook with me and would write down everything, especially when our platoon sergeant or our section leader would come in to meet with squad leaders to pass along orders. For example, if they told us about an inspection at 0700 hours the next morning, I'd write down the time and all the things they said our guys should have ready. I just didn't want to forget anything. Now, I was no ten-second Tom, the type of guy who forgets what was just said ten seconds after he's told something. There was just a lot going on, a lot of stuff was spinning in my head.

Don't forget, this was my first time leading a squad. My guys were counting on me to keep things straight and make sure that what I was bringing back from the platoon sergeant and section leaders was complete and accurate. Before I became a squad leader, I didn't feel the need to write as much down. Again, using inspections as an example, before my injury in Iraq, I might write down what I needed to bring for a particular inspection. But after Iraq, I would write, "Inspection, 0700 hours," and then the location, as well as everything we needed to bring.

We were scheduled to deploy in April, but the ash cloud that resulted from the eruptions of the Eyjafjallajökull volcano in Iceland that month wound up forcing the cancellation of tens of thousands of flights world-wide. So, we weren't going anywhere for a while.

One other thing happened before I left for Afghanistan, and it would figure into my life later in a very eerie way. My Uncle Toby, my mom's older brother, died from that overdose. As you might remember, he was my *real* father figure, not the worthless "sperm donor" Mike. Uncle Toby showed me how to work on cars, which came in handy with my 350Z. In fact, many times when my mom and I were getting into it, and I was running away like I told you earlier, I would wind up at Uncle Toby's. My uncle may not have always been the best role model. He'd been a junkie and was an alcoholic. But he eventually found God and cleaned himself up. I admired him for that. He had courage. Uncle Toby and I talked on the phone occasionally, and he did tell me that he was proud of me becoming a Marine. Sadly, he was exposed to the devastating side effects of a Fentanyl patch and passed away on April 17, 2010.

Because we were so close to departure, I didn't have time to get back and forth to Illinois for his funeral, which bothers me to this day. But then, in a way, I did see him. And I think it was one of the times in the hospital when I flatlined. But that would come later.

When we finally got the all clear a few weeks later, the families of my three guys came to see their Marines off. Betty was there. As we waited for buses that would take us to the airport, I went up to each of the families and introduced myself. I said, "I'm Corporal John Peck and I'm in charge of your Marine. I will make you a promise. I will get your Marine back in one piece."

Then we started the long journey from California to Maine and then from Maine to Kabul. A C130 transport plane brought us to Camp Leatherneck, the sprawling 1,600-acre base in the Helmand Province, about dead center in the southwest part of the country, and among the most dangerous locations.

Because this base had post exchanges, the couple of days we spent there were the final stop for any last-minute necessities or things like haircuts before we headed out to the much smaller—and not as well supplied—forward operating bases (FOB) where many of us would be stationed.

Once at our forward operating base, named Delhi, we did what we call a left-seat, right-seat kind of thing with the unit we were replacing. That's essentially where they give us the lay of the land (from the left seat), show-ing us the places not to go to, and what to be careful of in and around our area of operations. The U.S. surge against the Taliban was in full swing by then, with nearly 100,000 coalition troops in the country. And the Taliban was fighting back, including a rare ground attack on a NATO base in Kandahar.

Our base wasn't very big—maybe about 6,000 square feet. It wasn't Camp Leatherneck by a long shot, but it did have showers and a chow hall. We also had little squad bays, furnished with homemade tables and chairs left by the previous unit. Their main building material was Hesco barri-ers, which, you may remember, are collapsible wire-mesh containers—like chicken wire but on a much larger scale—and a thick fabric liner. The barri-ers can run six feet high and ninety-eight feet long and are great protection against blasts.

That was our home base for patrolling our area, which most often meant driving around the region. That turned out to be our main job. Now, for all the training we did as a mortar squad, just like in Iraq we never used our 81mm mortars while I was in Afghanistan. Part of the reason was the worries about potential collateral damage whenever you use an indirect fire weapon like a mortar or artillery. And, because of that issue, approvals to use the guns on any target would have to work themselves up the chain of command. And that just took too long.

Our platoon of about forty guys was divided up into two sections—each with four mortars, even though we weren't using them. Four of the mortar teams, including mine, stayed at our FOB, and the others were sent to a different base. The main mission, like I said, was to conduct patrols, be a presence, keep an eye out, and talk to the locals. We certainly got to know one local family, albeit quite unexpectedly. When we got to Afghanistan, we were riding around on mounted vehicles heading to the base where the first sergeant was located. We were driving along, and all of a sudden, the road gave way, and underneath was a waterway. Our vehicle fell into the ditch, and we couldn't get it out. So, we had no choice but to set up camp there and keep an eye on our vehicle. We were there for three long days before a military tow truck came to pull us out. As it turned out, we were stuck right in front of a guy's house. He and his family were very nice, and we talked a lot to him and his children. The one thing we didn't do is talk to his wife or daughters. There was one hard-and-fast rule we abided by in Afghanistan, and that was to never speak to a woman! Ever.

But my squad was less about patrolling and more about resupplying. They would send us to the other bases to deliver mail and drop off water and Meals Ready to Eat (MREs). We did that for about a month, making our rounds and then getting back to our base the same day or the next one. And once we were back, we'd just sit around and play cards, eat, and watch DVDs. It was cool in a way because we had the Internet and computers, and we could call our families and things like that. But it didn't take long to get tired of it. The guys were saying, "This is bullshit. We're just sitting around with our thumbs up our ass. We're not really doing anything."

One day, Doc Gould and I made idle conversation about what we'd do if we lost limbs. (Doc Gould was our Navy corpsman, and Marines often call their corpsmen Doc.) I told Gould I'd be okay if I lost my legs. I'd simply wheelchair around everywhere. But, I said, I'd be fucked if I lost my arms. And if I lost both my legs and arms, I'd want somebody to just shoot me on the spot. Doc Gould would remember that.

Meanwhile, we continued to get updates on other sections, and some of them were seeing action. Some were getting into firefights while out on patrol or when their bases would come under attack. Not every day, though. The attacks were sporadic in nature. And these were not major enemy assaults or anything like that. Not "Oh, my God, the shit is hitting the fan" kind of stuff, where you might have thirty or fifty guys attacking at one time. More like four-to-twelve enemy combatants. I mean, that's enough, but never like a battalion-sized assault. Again, these were sporadic.

The best way to describe it, from what we were told, was that our defenses were being tested. You know, people like to portray the enemy as being dumb, but they're not. This was Al-Qaeda, and they knew that a different battalion had come into their territory. They knew we were inexperienced and not used to the lay of the land or how things worked. This was their home turf, and we didn't know what we were doing in a lot of ways. So, all these little attacks were their way of testing us out, seeing if we're paying attention, and determining what we're capable of—how far we'll go when pushed.

But from my squad's point of view, all we're doing is driving around delivering MREs and water and mail while the other guys are taking fire and hitting improvised explosive devices (IEDs) and small arms fire—AK-47 kind of stuff usually, maybe a 9mm. But still, people at other bases were getting shot. A few guys were blown up. Some guys didn't make it.

And there we were sitting on our butts playing cards. We're asking, "Can we switch out with them? Can we do a tag team? Like two weeks of taxi service and then switch out and do two weeks of patrols?" That's what we kept pushing for, but we just kept getting turned down.

We didn't take any fire during that time. No small arms. No IEDs. No rocket-propelled grenades. Nothing. Honestly, it was just boring.

I know that's going to sound odd to most people, but you have to remember that we were infantry. We were the tip of the spear. I'm not going to say that we were the elite, because we weren't. But it was our job to go find the enemy and engage them. It was what we were trained to do.

The thing is, infantry guys aren't quite right in the head. And as you know by now, myself included. I don't mean we're brainwashed, or somehow seriously mentally ill. I mean we signed up for this job that required we go out and get shot at. That's what we were meant to do—and that's what we wanted to do. We wanted to find the enemy. We wanted to engage in firefights and be out there doing something. Look, we traveled 8,000 miles from California to Afghanistan. For what? To sit around and drive a damn MRAP? (That's military speak for a mine-resistant ambush-protected vehicle.) That's just a waste of our time and training.

Finally, we got a break from delivery service. Our first sergeant pulled us down to the base where he was stationed for a big company-sized movement through the area that would include machine gunners and sniper support. I wound up calling it the "death march." It had to have been a seven-kilometer or ten-kilometer march. We started in the morning, but it went late into the day before we were finally done.

The point was to engage the local population along the route and try to find out what kind of information they could, or would be willing to, share. Such as, has there been any kind of death threats? There were reports that the enemy was engaging some of our friendlies along this route, and the first sergeant wanted to make a point of showing our presence.

But, frankly, it was just ridiculous. At one point, on one of our breaks, Sergeant Ernie Mendez and I were maybe five meters apart. We took off our Kevlar and just looked at each other. We didn't have to say a word. We could see it in each other's faces: "What the fuck are we doing?" This guy, Mendez, he was built. This was not somebody you mess with. He had been in Fallujah and everything. But on this day, you could see the look: "Why are we doing this?"

It was bad. As I said, we were pushing 100 degrees. We had a lot of guys drop out. Guys in their prime. Zero body fat guys.

I ended up needing an IV. But the worst was yet to come. I lost my squad—my leadership post—that day. And ultimately that would lead to the worst day of my life.

Here's how it happened: A few days before the march, we had been given a list of the things we were supposed to bring along with us, including day packs, water, MREs, ammo, and the squad's M240 machine gun. I spread the word to my squad, but it turned out that Bulosan, our machine gunner, forgot his day pack. Fortunately, he could borrow one from another Marine who was not going out that day.

Unfortunately, he attached the thermal sight for the 240, an infrared sight that allows a shooter to see through smoke and fog, to the outside of the borrowed pack, using one of the straps.

About an hour and a half into the patrol, just before the sun came up, Bulosan approached me during a rest stop and said, "Corporal Peck, I lost the sight." I couldn't believe it. "Are you fucking serious?" "Yeah, I lost it," he repeated. I told him he needed to go see Sergeant Krumrie immediately and let him know what had happened. What I should have done next was radio the sergeant and let him know that Bulosan was headed his way and that we needed to halt the movement to find the damn thing. But I didn't. Big mistake on my part. Instead, I just assumed Bulosan had done as he was told and let it go at that.

Not long after, there was a security stop, and I checked in with Sergeant Krumrie in person to ask if Bulosan had gone to see him and reported what happened. "No," he replied. "What happened?" I then called Bulosan over to explain the loss of the sight. "What the fuck," I said. "Why didn't you tell him like I told you to?" His reply: "You never told me to tell him." I don't know if he was really surprised and hadn't heard me tell him to report to the sergeant, or if maybe he was hallucinating because of dehydration. Either way, this wasn't good. A thermal sight for the 240 was not something we wanted to fall into enemy hands.

Once back at the base, after I've had my IV, our section leader told me that Bulosan and I needed to sit separately and write statements to explain the loss of the sight. Some senior NCOs went over the statements and made the decision to relieve me of command.

I was crushed. I didn't feel any hostility towards the NCOs. I realized I made a terrible mistake, so I understood why they acted as they did. It boiled down to this: when Bulosan told me about the loss of the sight, I should have immediately notified Sergeant Krumrie so that we could have stopped and searched for it. By the time the sergeant found out, it was too late to go back and look for the sight. I spent the next few days thinking about what happened and what I should have done to prevent such a serious breach. It was not the best of times.

My squad was no longer. I was assigned to Sergeant Mendez. And because of all the shifting of personnel, Mendez's unit was short a person to handle the mine detector/sweeper—the guy who's out in front clearing the way for his fellow Marines. I volunteered. I was familiar with IEDs from my time in Iraq. I knew what patterns to look for, as well as about the assorted sizes and shapes. "There's no one better to trust as far as finding IEDs than me," I told Mendez. That boast, ironically, proved all too true.

By now, I'm down at the base where the first sergeant is, the place we started that ill-fated patrol. My unit was standing post at night and conducting patrols during the day. In other words, we're being utilized the way Marines are supposed to. Standing post is essentially standing guard. We kept watch day and night, 24/7, from four or five strategic positions on the base, each one armed with a machine gun, watching for enemy movement or anything unusual. The guys on post allow everyone else on base to be at least somewhat at ease.

Our patrols were no longer mounted. We were pushing into surrounding villages and communities on foot to introduce ourselves. Basically, what we were doing was telling the local population, "Hey, this is who we are. This is what we're doing here. This is what we're looking for." As the guy with the minesweeper, I was out front on these patrols. We walked from the base, sometimes taking the roads, but other times going through the fields to whatever village or compound was that day's destination.

A compound can essentially be a home, but it was usually a series of connected buildings. Typically in Afghanistan, the main rooms of a home—living room, dining area, and kitchen—aren't connected by hallways. You're going outside to go from room to room. And each compound will have a wall around it, with entry secured by a gate.

Upon our arrival, we'd knock. I know the movie version of our jobs is to kick doors down without warning and barge in, telling whoever is found inside to get on their knees and kiss the ground. We didn't do any of that. We knocked. And if someone was home and answered, we would tell them, through the interpreter who traveled with us, "Hey, we're Marines and we're here to help you. If you need anything, if you have anything damaged, we can help. If you have any Al-Qaeda leads, please come and talk to us. If you are receiving death threats, let us know about them and we'll find the person responsible. If you see something that you know isn't supposed to be happening, come and give us a heads-up."

If no one answered our knock, we needed permission from Lt. Saville before entering the house. I know, probably not the best thing in terms of respecting people's privacy. But we'd look through the rooms, as well as inspect the compound overall, inside and out, just to make sure there were no signs that anyone there was contributing to Al-Qaeda.

And that was our day. After our targeted destination had been checked out, and we'd had a chance to talk to the locals, we'd head back to the base. Every day, that's kind of what we did, back and forth. Each patrol might take five or six hours, maybe not even that sometimes. It all depended on where we were going. I don't think we ever visited the same place twice. We might pass a place that we'd already checked out on our way to somewhere else, but we didn't physically go back to a place once we'd inspected it.

Our days started early. We'd head out right after breakfast. It was pretty lax, though. We knew from orders usually received the night before—sometimes a few hours before—that we would be heading out and had a general time. These patrols were considered routine, not the kind of thing where you get five minutes notice, and they want you off the base checking something out. So, once you were up, the deal was, if you're hungry, eat something. Not the MREs, but those meals that are dehydrated and come in a bag. Just add water, and there's breakfast. They reminded me of some of those meals I had as a kid when my mom would be at work. Man, what I would have done for some of my Uncle Toby's special chili.

There could be anywhere from twenty to thirty guys per patrol. That's four or five fire teams. Nothing huge, but a well-armed patrol that could take care of itself. Now, if we had run into a battalion of terrorists, then maybe we might not be able to handle all that. But if approached by a squad of guys, we were good.

Figure each of us was carrying an M4. That's the shorter and lighter version (remember, lighter is always better humping all our gear in a hothouse like Iraq or Afghanistan) of the M16 that most people are familiar with. Other guys might have an M203, a 40mm grenade launcher that attaches to a rifle. Then others might have an M32, which is a grenade launcher with an ammo cartridge that makes the weapon look a bit like the Thompson submachine guns you see in old Al Capone movies. And likely someone in the group had a SAW, an M249 light machine gun.

The M249 can do some damage, putting out 650 rounds a minute. So, like I said, we're not up-armored ready for anything, but we do have the basics in terms of protection for a patrol. We can handle ourselves.

Out in front of all this firepower are two minesweepers. And one of those guys was me.

I know this might sound strange, but I was disappointed that nothing really happened in terms of engaging the enemy on these patrols. That was a letdown for me. Sick, right? But again, Marine infantry are kind of a sick breed. Plus, I was hell-bent on proving myself as a competent and capable Marine.

So, this was day-to-day life for me up until May 24.

Now, for most of these patrols, it's a meet-and-greet kind of thing. Just checking in with locals to introduce ourselves, get a feel for them, and get them a little comfortable with us. But sometimes, and that was the case on May 24, we were performing a routine patrol in a nearby village here to check out some sort of suspicious activity.

The village we targeted that day wasn't huge, maybe eight houses max. But they were all relatively close to one another, so we considered that a village. We divided the patrol evenly, with one group taking half the village to clear and the rest of us taking the other half. And we have all the basic patrol weaponry, plus on this day, I remember we had sniper support. In fact, on this particular day, Daniel Patterson, a buddy of mine, was the sniper and was watching us through his scope. So, while we were in close, the snipers had the bigger picture and were ready to provide cover fire if we missed something or maybe someone started coming at us from out of the blue.

There was one minesweeper per group, and we were taking one house, or compound, at a time. As usual, I wielded the sweeper in an arc, coming right up to the gate of a compound—and, of course, the sweeper would start picking up the metal in the gate. But I'd get as close as I could before I knew what was registering was the gate. From that point, we'd knock. Once inside, I continued sweeping. And my guys would follow behind, slowly, and very, very carefully. They weren't placing their steps exactly where mine had landed—like their right feet went precisely where my right foot was—but they were careful to stay within the arc of the sweeper. After I cleared an entrance, a few guys—always at least two—would go into each little area, whether the living room, dining room, or bedroom, checking for anything suspicious. We had gone through three of the four houses and found nothing. But it was the one thing we didn't find that really got our full attention: no one was home, in any of the houses. That might seem like a good thing. Fewer encounters mean less chance of an incident or danger, right? But, unfortunately, no people inside was not a good sign. There was probably a reason that there were no people or activity that morning; something was up.

The pattern continued for the last compound, where again I swept up to the gate. Now, technically, if no one is home, we're not supposed to be going in. But our first lieutenant gave the go-ahead. We knocked but got no reply. We entered, carefully, me sweeping and my guys following, on alert. I cleared each room, and they went in for further inspection. From the main rooms I went to the bathroom area. Nothing. Then I checked out a little storage hut, which was about three feet high. I went in, even getting down on my hands and knees to see if I could find anything. Again, nothing.

But while I was in the hut, a guy named Brian Johnson and our medic, Doc Gould, found some wires and a car battery in one of the rooms. In an empty house with no one around, this is very suspicious. Now we were really on edge.

While the rest of the guys were still inside, I figured I'd step outside and help pull security. I turned to let Sergeant Mendez know where I was headed and took one step forward.

That's when my life, at least as I knew it, changed forever.

With Daniel Patterson watching me through his scope, I stepped squarely on an IED. It didn't register right away; I swear to this day that the next thing I knew, it felt like I kicked myself in the head. And that might have been the last thing I felt.

As it was later described to me, the blast threw Sgt. Mendez to the ground and deafened him. He started screaming out our last names, hoping to hear from everyone. Johnson and Gould yelled back, but Mendez couldn't hear them. Then Johnson and Doc Gould realized I hadn't yelled back. They called out for me again. That's when they heard my groans.

There was a black cloud of soot and sand. Doc Gould started to run toward the blast crater. Johnson tried to stop him, warning of the danger of a secondary IED. "I don't care," Gould yelled and rushed to me.

He found both my legs blown off above the knee. My right arm just above the elbow was gone. My left arm was still attached, but the skin from the middle of my forearm to my fingers had been peeled back. Degloved, they call it.

Marines carry tourniquets on patrol, so they began putting them on my legs and arms. I screamed they were hurting me, but Johnson slapped me and said, "Stop being such a little bitch."

All I remember was that my eyes were caked with dust and black soot. I couldn't see or hear anything. I remember these black figures hovering over me. I saw four of them. They're working on me. *Something's seriously wrong,* I thought to myself, as I was going in and out of consciousness. At some point, I'm told, Lt. Saville arrived, and I asked him if my family jewels were still there. He said they were.

But I couldn't do anything. I couldn't lift anything. I couldn't move. I felt nothing.

I somehow managed to say—I actually thought it was just in my head, but apparently I was saying it out loud—"Don't let me die in this fucking hellhole. I don't want to die here. I can't die here."

I kept saying it. Constantly. At least that's all I thought I was saying.

Next thing I know, I blacked out. *This is it,* I thought.

But I came back to, and it felt like I was being carried; I felt weightless. Then I could feel the intense gusts of the rotor wash of a helicopter hitting me. And then I'm inside it. Things don't go dark, really, but I can tell I'm being put inside the medevac chopper. At least that's what it felt like was happening. Then there was one more shape above me. "Hey, you're gonna go to sleep for a little bit," the man said.

Before I went out, though, I clearly remember looking back at my guys. They were everything to me, and now I'm letting them down. "I'll see you later," I yelled at them. "See you in a few more days. I'll be back, boys."

As I learned later, as the chopper lifted off, Doc Gould watched it leave and felt a shiver of guilt. He remembered what I said earlier. He was supposed to shoot me.

TWELVE

WAKING UP WITHOUT ARMS AND LEGS

I WAS GONE, BLACKED OUT. I LATER LEARNED IT WAS FOR THE BETTER PART OF three months, with only rare spells of lucidity.

Initially, I was taken to Bagram Air Force Base, in the eastern part of the country. Bagram is near an ancient city of the same name, in the Parwan Province. The hospital—the Heathe N. Craig Joint Theater Hospital—is as good as any in the States, and the docs there have saved countless guys' lives, just like mine. I can't recall ever being conscious at Bagram.

A doctor told me recently that at some point on the flight from Bagram to the U.S. military hospital in Germany, I came to and spoke to him. I don't remember it, but he told me that I wanted to know how bad my injury was, and his reply was, "Really messed up." What I didn't realize at the time was that really messed up meant that I was missing both of my legs and one of my arms. He told me that I was saying that I wanted to die. "Don't let me live," I told him and anyone else who was listening. "Please just go ahead and kill me."

Obviously, they didn't. In fact, I coded a few times—meaning my vital signs dropped to dangerously low levels—and they fought hard to keep me alive.

God only knows what was going on in my head then. During one of the times I was seriously out, there he was—Uncle Toby. Dead or not, he

84

appeared to me, with his trademark smirk. We had this nice, short talk. He told me, "John, you can't quit. You can't give up. You need to go back down there and give them hell." And that was it. I don't know if it was the drugs or my hallucinations or what, but I swear I saw him that one last time. He somehow gave me the strength to deal with the nightmare that was ahead.

But the truth is that even though we were prepared for what we would face in combat, nothing, absolutely nothing, can prepare you for being blown up and losing your arms and legs.

From May 24, the day I stepped on that IED in Afghanistan, until the day in September when they moved me out of intensive care and I was no longer medically sedated, my fate was entirely in the hands of other people. No longer was I the strong Marine in charge; I was broken. Literally.

Basically, during all those surgeries and painkillers and the hours and hours of care, the doctors and nurses were trying to figure out, day to day, the answer to this simple question: can we pull this guy through? And, yeah, they figured it out. They could—and would—save me from the trauma of a blast that took away three limbs and, later, a flesh-eating fungus that, in some ways, was equally bad. In fact, I later learned that only two Marines had ever survived this horrible organism—Sgt. Maj. Ray Mackey and me. That's a distinction I can live without.

But the question now became: okay, they could save me, but for what? What could I do in this condition? And only I could answer that.

Of course, I have no recollection of what happened to me from the time I was in Germany in the hospital to when I returned to the states. I was medically sedated. I had to rely on primarily my mom, and to a lesser extent Betty, to piece together the first few months. According to my mom, she received a call from Gene that I was in Germany and undergoing treatments there. That's all she knew at the time. She was told they put me on a plane, and I was expected to arrive in Bethesda on a Friday. But as my mom was picked up at the airport to meet me at the hospital, she overheard an officer say, "Yes, she's here with me now." That freaked her out. He gently explained to my mom that my plane was diverted to Newfoundland, Canada. Apparently, my blood pressure had dropped dramatically during the flight, and to be safe rather than sorry, they wanted to get me somewhere fast to get stabilized.

My mom was terrified that my injuries were causing me to bleed out on the plane. And she should know, since by that time, she was in the medical field for more than thirty years. I arrived on Sunday at Bethesda. They told my family that I was finally stabilized. My mom met the ambulance; she was horrified!

"I looked at John and he was sweating," my mom said. "I took his hand and whispered in his ear, 'John, I'm here and we're going to do everything we can to get through this, but you need to fight.'"

Not only was I sweating, but my mom felt my forehead, and she knew I was running a high fever. At one point, she told me that it was up to 106 degrees. What caused the fever was that damn flesh-eating fungus—aspergillus is its name—but at the time they didn't know that. The Centers for Disease Control and Prevention defines the fungus as a common mold that lives both indoors and outdoors; however, there are different types of the fungus—some mild and other more serious. People who have weakened immune systems, like I did after the blast, are at a higher risk of developing severe medical problems—sometimes so severe they lead to death.

The medical personnel had me all covered up under four thick blankets. With my mom's medical training, she knew that someone with a high fever should never be covered up that heavily. So, my mom pulled the covers off, and from what she told me, the medical folks in the ambulance were—how should I say—completely annoyed with my mom's trying to take over. She told me she said something to them like, "Don't tell me what's right for my son; I'm his mom."

As any of my wounded warrior friends whose moms came to Bethesda to take care of them know, don't mess with a mamma grizzly. Once the doctors got a closer look at me, they told my mom she was right-on and took me immediately to surgery to clean up my wounds.

The next day, I was under heavy sedation to manage my excruciating pain. My mom and wife would be there at my side every day; my mom took charge. No surprise there. She literally checked all of my wounds and every part of my body many times a day. "The truth is that nurses can do only so much with such a huge patient load, and it's hard to take care of all those patients' needs, which is totally understandable," my mom said. "When you have a mom there it can make a difference. I made sure I was the one to give John a bath, because I could see what was going on and take any action if I needed." And since I was out of it, man was I glad my mom was around.

Oh, and one other thing. You may have noticed above that I lost *three* limbs to the blast. What about the fourth? Well, after I arrived at Bethesda from Canada, Betty noticed that the little finger on my left hand had turned blue. The surgical team at Bethesda then discovered that I had no circulation at all in my left arm; the arterial stent that had been placed there had collapsed. After considering the bum stent and the trauma to the arm from the IED—the "degloving"—the surgeons made the decision to remove my left arm. Betty signed off on it.

I was now officially a quadruple amputee.

I was medically sedated—basically unconscious—for three months, from the end of May through August. A couple of months before I fully woke up, I contracted pneumonia, apparently from being on a respirator for so long. Luckily, my mom was keeping a daily journal, and that was helpful to me in so many ways, though at the time I had no idea why. I don't know what I would have done without my mom by my side once again. She took the lead in making sure I was being taken care of properly; she was the person to talk with the doctors because of her medical training. What most people don't realize is that even though wounded warriors get the best care in the world, in my opinion, things can still go terribly wrong. Someone, even with the best intentions, can miss a vital sign, give you the wrong pill, or not notice something that only a mother can. Having my mom serve as my advocate when I was not able—I think it was critical to my recovery. But despite everyone's best efforts, and as if the pneumonia weren't bad enough, the aspergillus fungus was busy invading my body.

The doctors occasionally gave me what they called a "sedation holiday," meaning they would take me off some of the most powerful drugs to give my body a break. I was on, at one time or another, morphine, dilaudid, and ketamine. Taking me off those drugs was no holiday, believe me. The pain was intense. But the holidays did make me lucid for brief moments. For those moments of clarity, if you can call them that, my mom would ask me questions and tell me to shake my head one time if the answer was a "Yes."

"I asked you if you realized how badly you were hurt," my mom told me after I was fully conscious. "John, did you know that you lost your arms and legs?" she said. "You shook your head, which meant, 'Yes.' Then she told me, "John, do you know one of the positive things about your injuries?" I apparently crinkled my nose a bit. "Well, John," she said, "You finally got rid of those long, hairy toes!" I guess I thought that was funny because I smiled for a second, then went right back to sleep.

I continued my drugged-out unconscious, briefly conscious life through the summer. Meanwhile, the doctors were doing everything they could to manage my flesh wounds, but they still managed to get infected. My mom noticed and pointed it out to the doctors and nurses. You need to do something, and fast, she told them. They did a biopsy and—sure enough—discovered I had been infected with this toxic fungus aspergillus. They told my mom and wife that if the infection reached my abdomen and bloodstream, it would likely be fatal. That's what a killer that damn fungus is.

"This was devasting news," my mom told me later, recalling the worst of the fungus scare. "The doctors told us that we needed to spend as much time with you as we could and said we may want to bring the family to the hospital just in case we needed to make some end-of-life decisions."

That meeting changed everything for my mom. There were two staff sergeants there, three therapists, and one chaplain—all trying to explain, in the gentlest way possible—the probability that I was going to die. My mom tried not to interrupt them, but you can't ever keep her down. She told them not to sugarcoat my situation and tell it like it was. "I realize that they do sugarcoat the bad news to protect a patient's family, but it made it harder for me because I knew what they were saying; I just wanted to hear the down and dirty," my mom explained.

After that, they asked my family if they needed anything and gave them some time to talk and think about what to do. They closed the room off so my mom, her dad, and Gene could confer. She also asked the doctors during the meeting if they could give them some more time for the rest of the family to get there, just in case I didn't make it.

It was unbelievable what happened next, according to my mom. The Marines sent police officers to our house in Antioch, picked up both of Gene's daughters from work, then drove them back to the house. A state trooper was waiting and told them to pack their bags. The trooper drove them to the airport with lights and sirens blazing. Believe it or not, the officer initially got in trouble for doing that but later was vindicated. The next day, everyone was assembled at the hospital, including Betty's parents, who came to support her.

"We were in a state of him living second to second most of that July," my mom said. I'm sure she was beyond tired and emotionally spent. "They took him into surgery for a wound debridement (a procedure that includes the removal of necrotic tissue) on July Fourth. Finally, around the third week of July, John was beginning to fight the infection. Which was good."

It was a hard time for everyone, especially my mom. There was a lot of family drama, medical ups and downs, but in the end, there was lots of love. I vaguely remember—or maybe recall from what my mom told me—that she would sit with me in the hospital before I was completely awake and tell me stories and even sing songs. "I'm not the biggest fan of country music, but I know John loved the Billy Ray Cyrus song, 'Achy, Breaky Heart,' my mom said. "I would put earbuds in the iPod and put one bud in John's ear and the other in mine, and I would sing that song to him. It was like doing a car dance in the hospital. And even though my brother Toby had passed, John kept asking for him over and over when he was finally able to speak."

My room at the hospital, incidentally, was the best decorated on the ward. My wife had put up a large clipboard and attached tons of photos. I had these two big windows, maybe four feet by five feet, that you couldn't look out because there were so many get-well cards taped to them. A lot were from folks back in Antioch. Actually, I found out they held a fund drive in my hometown and raised about $70,000 to pay for my family's travel costs and other expenses.

But the effects of the blast were constantly with me, in all kinds of unexpected ways. For example, during one of my sedation holidays, I had a trach inserted into my throat. But before they could remove it, they had to insert a small camera into the hole in my throat and have me eat or drink something. That way, they could make sure things were going down the throat properly. They also inserted this little device that allowed me to talk.

When I failed the first test at swallowing, I asked for something to drink. During this whole trachea period, I couldn't drink anything. I was allowed to have ice chips, but only so many at a time. Betty would sometimes sneak me some extras. The only way I got real liquid was through a feeding tube in my nose. I hated that damn tube!

In fact, after that first swallowing test failure, I begged the nurse for some Mountain Dew. All I got was some vague promise. "Maybe next time, John," she told me. But then another nurse came into my room holding two cans. I started in on her about the Mountain Dew, and we kidded awhile. She poured the first out somewhere (I couldn't move my head to see) and left the second on my bedside table. "Hey, that's a Mountain Dew, and I'm gonna figure out a way to drink it," I told her. Turns out it wasn't Mountain Dew at all—only the gunk they poured down my feeding tube! So much for the power of persuasion. But despite a few moments like that, it was a terrifying moment when it really hit me that I was now another grim statistic of the War on Terror. I joined the small, but exclusive group of guys missing both of their arms and legs. Welcome to the quadruple amputee club!

By September 2010, I had been transferred from Bethesda Naval Hospital to the old Walter Reed Army Hospital in Washington, D.C., and though I was still on pain meds, I was conscious and somewhat alert. This was before the two facilities were merged to create the new Walter Reed National Military Medical Center, on the old Bethesda campus.

Sadly, my mom was no longer taking care of me. It's a long story, but suffice to say that there was friction between my mom and Betty. Since she was my wife, Betty was the one making all the decisions related to my health and in general. That's when Betty decided to tell me lies about my mom so I would take her side and not my mom's. One of those lies was when Betty said that my mom would instruct her dog, Bailey, to be aggressive to Betty in an effort to scare her. I'm not completely sure to this day why Betty felt the need to bad-mouth my mom. It was probably a control issue. To my discredit, I believed Betty. So much so that I told my mom that she should go home to Illinois. It was ugly. I actually scolded my mom, telling her that I would have base security remove her if she didn't leave. Like I said, my mom and I have a habit of bumping heads. But it still bothers me to this day that I was so belligerent. Having endured so much pain, being on a massive number of drugs, plus the trauma of the blast, affected my personality and not always for the better. The truth was I thought I was protecting my wife, and I believed her.

So, Betty and her mom stayed with me, but it was no picnic. The old Walter Reed was not in the best section of the city, and it still had some of the conditions made public in a 2007 investigation by the *Washington Post*, like mice droppings, black mold, and other shit. (It was officially closed in 2011.) But at that point, I didn't care. I remember thinking to myself that I felt weird because I still had no clothes on, and for someone used to wearing a uniform and carrying more than one hundred pounds on his back—well, that was strange. But, at least I was awake and cognizant. My skin felt very prickly and was incredibly sensitive to touch, so most of the time I was happy to be totally naked. When they needed to move me, they simply threw a sheet over me, and I was good to go.

I heard several reasons from the doctors for this skin sensitivity. Some said that I wasn't touched and rolled around enough while I was sedated, and so my skin just got hypersensitive to anything and everything. But then I also heard that it might have been a side effect of the medication for the fungus. Either way, here's what I knew for sure: if someone laid a hand on me, anywhere on my body except my face—even if it were the most loving, gentle touch on my shoulder—I would scream in pain. Intense agony. I'm not even sure I can describe how bad it was anymore. In one way, it was kind of like when your foot falls asleep, and you get that pins-and-needles feeling. But that's almost funny, right? This wasn't funny at all. This shit hurt. It was the bizarre pins-and-needles sensitivity combined with an intense burning sensation. And all this was going on when I was still on methadone, which is a powerful, serious painkiller. Even that wasn't enough to keep me from going into spasms of agony when anyone touched me.

The other thing I vividly remember from this point was that I couldn't even lift up what was left of my arms. Same with my legs. I was like a board. Know what my therapist called me? Her little "wooden plank." Yeah, that was her nickname for me. I had no range of motion. Zero. I felt helpless. You know how magicians have that trick where they place the assistant in a box and tell them not to move? I would've been perfect for that.

Once I settled in at Walter Reed, they decided I should start therapy as soon as possible, both physical and occupational. The physical therapy was to get the body I had left to become more mobile, stretching it out, helping me regain muscle strength, and pushing me to figure out how far I could go. In combination with that, occupational therapy was the preparation for me someday using prosthetic limbs and relearning tasks for basic daily living.

At that point, people couldn't come into my room without being gowned up in those yellow paper smocks, with gloves and masks. After the fungus, the doctors were still worried about what I might have in my system and my ability to withstand infection. It had been the same way in Bethesda and carried over at Walter Reed. For any wounded warrior, especially someone suffering from the loss of all four limbs, daily life is exhausting and unrelenting. Every day, I would have to endure hours and hours of physical and occupational therapy. Countless doctor visits and endless tests. I had to not only get over the deadly fungus, but heal all of my internal injuries. I had a hernia, tinnitus, the single head of my left bicep was consumed by fungus, and the first layer of my abdominal muscle—fasciitis—was also eaten away. Plus, the blast blew off my limbs—not in clean cuts like some of the other guys—but jagged sections of torn flesh. It wasn't pretty. The doctors and staff came up with a comprehensive therapy plan for me. They said it would take some time—years in fact—for me to become semi-independent. And when you are feeling so helpless and vulnerable, having people around you who are kind and patient can make all the difference. In my case, that would be Kyla.

For my first therapy session, two gowned-up therapists came to my room and introduced themselves. The woman said her name was Kyla and she was going to be my physical therapist—yes, this is the woman who would eventually be calling me her "little plank." That was what we wounded warriors affectionately call "amputee humor."

I liked Kyla from the start. She was in her mid-thirties and was from Pennsylvania. She had dark, wavy hair and a way of looking at you that made you feel comfortable. She also had this wicked sense of humor. Over time, she would be the one I could confide in, no matter how dark my thoughts. And they would get dark.

There was also guy named Orin who would be the one to handle my occupational therapy. They explained their roles and what their jobs entailed, telling me what they were going to do and how they would help me. On the surface, my attitude was, sure, whatever. Remember I was still heavily medicated at this point. I was agreeable to just about anything. But another part of me, from the time I could really comprehend what had happened and how extensive my injuries were, had thought, okay, this is all part of the deal and I have to get used to certain things. But truthfully, there is nothing that can prepare someone mentally or physically to wake up and not be able to touch your face or walk to the bathroom. Or to watch yellow pus come out of my arms when Orin stretched and massaged them. (He called it yellow pudding. Never again will I eat pudding.)

As I listened to them explain how they were going to get me ready to use prosthetics, and through our sessions learn how to be more independent, I felt sick to my stomach. I was skeptical, to say the least. I don't know if I raised my doubts then, or on another day, but I couldn't help but think, *Guys, I'm in a hospital bed. I don't have arms or legs. I can't move any part of my body. How the hell are you guys going to help me? What the hell am I going to do? How am I ever going to be independent again?*

I was not their first amputee wounded warrior, so they understood where I was coming from. They very patiently explained that with the use of prosthetics, I would gradually be able to become more and more independent. I would discover ways to do things for myself like comb my hair, cook a meal, or take a shower without the humiliation of having someone there to wash those areas I can't reach with my stubs. Eventually, they assured me, I would even be able to live alone; there was nothing I could do at that point to challenge what they were saying. But when you have suffered the type of trauma I have—losing both my arms and legs—it was tough to believe that I would return to my previous independent lifestyle. But I guess these guys know what they are doing. After all, the DoD in 2016 estimated that 1,650 service members had lost limbs and were using prosthetics. So, they have lots of experience with these devices, and working with guys like me. I wish their comforting words had resonated a little more with me.

I wasn't saying "no." It wasn't like I had a choice when it came to therapy—but, truthfully, I was thinking, *Really, guys? Seriously?* Now, part of me knew that certain things were possible. I couldn't quite get it for myself, but I had seen and talked to other wounded warriors during their recovery process. In fact, there were some guys who had less serious injuries than mine and were in worse shape mentally. I made it my mission after I began to feel better to visit them and try to give them a pep talk. In fact, I found out that Daniel Patterson, the same guy who watched me get blown up through his sniper scope, was now at Walter Reed. He stepped on an IED and lost both legs. I went to see him and gave him a Nintendo 3DS that someone had sent me. I told him to let me know if he needed anything. He had a trach tube in his mouth and couldn't say anything, but he gave me a big smile. That helped. I think one of the best ways to help yourself recover is by reaching out to others facing similar horrific injuries. I was always the type of person who wanted to help other people, but this time it was personal. I felt their pain. I knew what it was like to lose your limbs. I saw relationships fall apart. I now had a new mission.

Then there was Todd Nicely, who, like me, is one of five quadruple amputees from the wars in Iraq and Afghanistan. He started to come to my room for visits while I was still in Bethesda. He was already walking on his prosthetic legs. *Okay*, I thought when I saw him. *Maybe there is some hope here for me, and maybe I'll be able to walk again.* But one of the things I noticed was that Todd had both of his leg "nubs." (That's what we call what's left of our arms and legs. The medical term is "residual limbs.") But I had a hip disarticulation, which means the cut on one leg was very high—right up to my hip. That's a major difference when it comes to having something to attach to a prosthetic device. That's why, other than some preliminary work, I would never really use prosthetic legs.

(Let me also say one thing about prosthetics. I think some folks believe that once a warrior gets prosthetic arms or legs, everything is cool. It's not. Even with the better fits, wearing prosthetic legs can be incredibly painful and uncomfortable for what's left of the warrior's leg. Plus, you expend about 200 percent more energy to walk with them. So after even a brief walk, you can be exhausted and in a lot of pain.)

Another difference had to do with my arms. All my fellow quads have one arm amputated above the elbow and one below. The thing is, though, in my arm with the elbow, I don't have a bicep. And your bicep is what allows you to bend your elbow. Think about the muscle that moves when you're doing curls. Well, the flesh-eating fungus essentially ate my bicep. So, the radial muscles in my forearm had to compensate. Just another setback for me. So, yes, we can draw hope from one another's stories, but even the quads have differences that make each person's recovery very different from any other. Still, I have to say I always really enjoyed talking to Todd. He would let me ask all kinds of questions about my recovery and gave me pointers about his. I wish I could remember them all, but I was heavily medicated during that time, so not all of it sank in.

Another regular visitor and source of hope was Tyler Southern, who would come by with his then-fiancée, who is now his wife. Tyler is a triple amputee. When he started visiting, I still couldn't lift my arms or legs. My arms felt like they were glued to my side. I could barely move my head from side to side. But one day, Tyler came in, and I had this huge smile on my face. He saw it and said, "Dude, why are you smiling like that? You're creeping me out."

I said, "Look what I can do." I start doing this awkward wiggling motion, and he finally says, "Are you having a seizure?" And I was like, "No, no, no. Look, I'm moving my arms. I'm moving my arms."

We both just start cracking up. Tyler said, "John, you lifted your arm about a centimeter. Are you seriously happy about that?" "Hell, yeah, I am," I shot back.

I had been working on it for a few days, too. For a guy who felt trapped in a body that wasn't responding to his desires to move, a centimeter was a lot. I felt happy for the first time in a long while.

So, that's what Kyla and Orin had to work with. They saw a guy who was desperate to gain back some mobility and see what was going to come next in life, versus a guy who was having a tough time imagining if he'd ever even be able to get out of his hospital bed. But there is something genetically in me that has always kicked in when I needed it the most. It's like having DNA that constantly is telling you to pick yourself up and never give up. I could and would not accept the fact that I was a now a quadruple amputee. Of course, I knew I was. But I had a goal, and that was to be able to be independent again and do something meaningful with my life. I've always pushed through pain—emotional and physical—and this was no exception.

I'm not going to lie; I also have my bad days. I'm a Marine, for God's sake. And even though this period was among the most challenging I have ever experienced, I had to summon up that inner strength once again.

I don't know how many sessions we had in my room before we switched to what we called MATC—the Military Advance Training Center—where all the wounded warriors did their physical therapy. I do remember, though, that I still wasn't wearing any clothes when we started going down there. They had to cover my entire body with just a sheet. So basically, I'm like Tarzan with a little fricking loincloth on. Also, anyone coming into contact with me still had to "gown up" and wear the hair nets and surgical masks.

I traveled by gurney to get to MATC. To transfer me from my bed, they had to put a sheet underneath me, lift me up, and then put me down on the gurney. It was pure agony! They did it gently, but it was the most painful thing because my skin was so sensitive. It was just horrible. Once I got there, I had to be transferred again, this time to a workout mat. Not one that just lay flat on the floor, though. Picture something about the size of a queen mattress that can be raised or lowered, so the therapist doesn't have to keep bending over to work with someone. And while the mats were mattress size, they were not padded in the same way. There was some padding, but it was mostly hard. It was also covered with a clean sheet that they changed for each guy they worked on.

To start, the sessions were easy and relaxed, about a half hour each day. That was about twice as long as the sessions in my room, but the one similarity was that the focus was on stretching. The therapists would tell me what the plan was for that day and remind me of their goals and what they thought I needed. They started off by running their hands over me very lightly because of my skin sensitivity. Not quite like patting me down, but just a gentle way of getting me used to being touched. And they even got into some stretching early on. This wasn't "Let's push and see if he can raise his arm over his head." I had zero range of motion, so it was more like "Let's see if we can get your arm slightly off the mat, just enough to see if we can slide a piece of paper underneath."

Of course, if getting lifted by a sheet was painful, so was their touch, even though they were very light about it. They knew about my pain and they were trying to be soft and loving, but they still had jobs to do. The idea was that eventually, my skin would get used to being touched again. Basically, it was up to me to suck it up. They were being as careful as possible, but they couldn't do therapy without touching me. And part of therapy is moving once-immobile limbs a little more each day, so there is pain from that on top of the skin sensitivity.

While sucking it up, though, I still had a few choice words for them. Sometimes I tried very hard to be polite. I'd say, "Please stop, you're hurting me." Other times, the pain was so unbearable, I'd have tears coming out of my eyes and would scream, "Stop! Stop! You're hurting me. I hate you. I fucking hate you." Now Kyla, who was working on my arms, would stop at times like that. She was the sweet one. But Sgt. Webb—the therapist who replaced Orin after a short time—she had charge of my legs, and she was a brute. She would seriously challenge me.

The point is to push you, a little further each time. Maybe they get you to extend your arm beyond what you think you are capable of. Next time they push a little more until there's pain. They see what you can bear, and then they'll hold that limb there for a few seconds—sometimes a few seconds too long because I'd have to say, "That's enough." I can't say I fully understood everything that was going on—I was still on a lot of meds, don't forget—but I accepted it. If I wasn't wholeheartedly into it, I was at least going along.

The agonizing stretching and skin touching lasted for months. During that time, Kyla wanted me to come down to MATC in a gurney chair, which is a chair that lie flat but can increase the angle at which you lie, eventually getting you to sit upright. This was the only way, Kyla said, to stretch my back. When I finally got to the point where I could lift my own arms, even just a millimeter off the bed, we moved to the next level. There was no letting up. They would strap what we called resistance bands around my arms or my legs, and I'd try to fight back and raise my arms despite the bands. They came in a series of colors, with each color signifying a different level of resistance. Maybe red was easy, blue a little harder, yellow medium, and black "death." Once they could see I was getting stronger, I graduated from the bands to sandbag weights that they would attach to my arms with Velcro.

The first time we tried the weights, I was able to lift a whopping five pounds. It's not something I'm proud of. Before the injury, I could easily lift one hundred twenty pounds, and here I was hoping to lift a measly five? It was embarrassing Then again, before the blast I was over six feet tall, two hundred five pounds, with maybe 3-to-5 percent body fat mass index. In the hospital, I got down to ninety pounds; you could play the xylophone on my rib cage. That's no exaggeration. I think I may have even dropped below ninety pounds.

At the same time as I was starting on the weights, they were also giving me other exercises to do. One involved a cylindrical object that they would place under my nubs, and I'd push off that to lift my butt off the table. I'd use the same thing on my sides as well, though less so on my left side. That's my most sensitive side—pure bone with no cushioning, so it's harder for me to lie on that side, even today. The pain was not like before, when I would scream, "Don't touch me; don't touch me." But it still smarted.

Overall, though, the sensitivity largely went away after a few months of touching and therapy. But during that time, the doctors discovered another terrible result of the flesh-eating fungus. One day, during occupational therapy, to help me sit up, the therapist would wrap a towel around my back and try to pull me up. I was having the hardest time with it and certainly couldn't do it on my own. So, they checked me out and discovered that I was missing the first layer of my abdominal muscles. All from the fungus. Usually, if the fungus has infected a part of the body, the only way to remove it is to cut it out. That's what had happened with parts of my left leg and arm. But you couldn't do that with my abs. There was no way, so instead, they bombarded me with antibiotics. It's gone now, but to this day I can't do a proper sit-up. I'd eventually learn to sit up on my own, but that came much later.

While the physical side of recovering was grueling and painful, it was no match for the emotional side of things.

My first trip outside the hospital was for my birthday, September 13. I got to go off-base with my wife, a friend of hers, and another Marine. It was a wonderful day. We rented a wheelchair and headed to Red Lobster and had a seafood feast. Afterward, we went to see the movie "Resident Evil: Afterlife," which had just come out. And, of course, just like in the hospital, I couldn't do anything for myself. I needed help. I couldn't move my arms, and someone had to feed me, which was humiliating. I was wearing this loose t-shirt because of the skin thing. Clothes still bothered me, but it's not like I could go out naked. I looked like a mess, and I was in horrible shape overall. If people were staring or having any problems with me being there, I was oblivious to it. I was so totally focused on myself. It was like, "Oh, my God, somewhere else besides the fricking hospital." I was in bliss, and just totally in the moment of being out and trying to do something normal. I felt free for the first time in a very long while.

But that didn't last long.

Maybe a week or two later, I started talking to my wife about her returning to California to pick up her stuff and to maybe get my car and bring it back, too. She was totally agreeable, and we bought her a ticket and off she went. But, as I would discover, her idea of the trip was entirely different.

While Betty was in California, and with my mom gone, Betty's mom stayed with me. They gave her a place to sleep at the ward. They had a chair there for her that folded out, basically like a big recliner. While she was my mother-in-law, we weren't all that close. She was a quiet, middle-aged lady from New Hampshire; we had zero in common, especially with me in my current shape. She did try to be helpful in her own way, though. If I needed something from the small room on the ward that had snacks and drinks, she would get them for me. If I felt too warm, she would remove one of my blankets. There was no question that she was good-natured and kind. And I really did try to be pleasant to her, as well. But even though Betty's mom was there to help me, her mere presence started to make me feel like I had betrayed my mom. You have to realize that when you have faced such a devastating injury as mine, plus also having a TBI, and being loaded up with pain meds, you are not yourself. I felt vulnerable and alone.

A week went by, and I still didn't hear anything from my wife. And with no hands, it's not like I can pick up the phone and call whenever I like. Finally, I asked her mom to dial Betty's number on my phone. Our initial conversations were bad. Really bad, in fact. She wanted to know why I hadn't called her. "Hey, I have no hands. I couldn't call you," I told her.

From there, things went from bad to worse. It turns out she didn't want to come back to Washington but wanted to start taking criminal justice classes out there in California. I was shocked! I had a Marine buddy do a little investigating about what colleges were near her in California and which offered those courses. There weren't many, so I asked her, "Why can't you come back and go to school here in D.C.?"

That was only the beginning of my marital nightmare. For my injuries, I got $100,000 from insurance. I found out soon that about $30,000 of it was already gone. It turns out that Betty took it out of my account, claiming she needed the money for "retail therapy." What the hell is that? Here I am with no arms and legs and suffering, and she's in La La land shopping! I also discovered some huge bar bills, expensive dinners—that kind of thing. And while she was with me at the hospital, she took to wearing very skimpy dresses, which I guess she bought as part of her so-called retail therapy. Worse, she was flirting like crazy with other Marines. (In fact, if you can believe it, I later found out she was actually sexting her new boyfriend in California while she was sitting right next to me in the hospital.)

On one of my last calls to Betty when she was in California, I just told her, "Look, I need you here. If you aren't by my side, helping me through all this, you aren't my wife." I told her that if she couldn't come back and support me, both mentally and physically, then we needed to get a divorce.

Sad to say, she agreed. She said some other things during that time that hurt me more than words could ever say. She said to me in the coldest way possible, "You're disgusting; no one will ever love you." Okay, I wasn't the same physically fit guy she married, but that doesn't mean I was worthless. I remember just lying there in bed sobbing. It was probably among the three most devasting times of my life so far. Mike abandoning me, losing my memory and all four of my limbs, and now this. In fact, her reaction to me after my second injury was cruel. I had no idea how I was going to survive. The triple A's, as I call them, were on full display—abuse, abandonment, and abrogation. I felt helpless and hopeless.

Even though I was making so much progress in my physical therapy sessions, what Betty said put me right back into my dark spot. I was afraid of what I would become. What would my life be like as a quadruple amputee? Would I ever find love again? Could I ever trust another woman? These were only a fraction of the thoughts that consumed me as my hospital stay progressed.

Over the next couple of months, Betty made it perfectly clear that she wasn't there for me. Plus, the havoc she caused between my mom and me was terrible She turned out to be someone I didn't recognize. I guess that's the luck of the draw. But with my injuries and now marital problems, my insecurity was growing by the day.

The other thing that got me down was that my mom was gone. Betty sowed the seeds of doubt in me, and it left its scars. As a result of Betty's lies, my mom needed to regroup and recover herself. She spent a few days in the hospital, and that did her good. But she had to return to work and get back to her own life. I felt badly that I believed Betty's lies about my mom, but I learned an important lesson. And that was never trust someone implicitly, unless they earned that trust. It was like what Ronald Reagan said during the Cold War—"Trust but verify." My mom was there for me for my entire life, and it pains me now to think what I did to her. You never really appreciate things until they're gone. But the sad fact was that I didn't always appreciate my mom, and now that she left, I was completely alone and afraid.

So now, just four months after getting blown up, and on top of everything else that's going on, I'm heartbroken. And all the back-and-forth that divorce entails just kept making things worse. Betty's mom tried to blame things on one of Betty's friends, but I knew better. I told her mom that it was probably best that she leave. Thankfully, she agreed. Now I was truly alone.

* * * *

Obviously, all of this really put me on a downward spiral mentally—down into what I would call my "dark spot." I had been blown up in the spring and here it was fall, just four or five months later. No wife; no life. Despite everything, I hadn't even considered suicide before. My attitude from the start was that no matter how screwed up things were, I was going to own this problem. I was going to figure this out, whatever it took. I guess it was Marine training and childhood survival skills that kicked into high gear.

But the dark spot kept getting bigger.

I began to seriously contemplate killing myself. What did I have to live for? Who would ever love me again? In my despair, I figured out how a guy with no arms and legs, who wasn't even able to feed himself, could do it. This would be the one and only time my core will to survive—to overcome, to move ahead—would waver.

At the end of my hallway was a doorway leading to a flight of stairs. From the stairs side, to enter the hallway, there was a conventional latch that a person would need hands to be able to open. But from the hallway side—my side—there was a push bar. Press on that, the door opens, and the stairs await. So, my plan was that I would ram my chair through the door and throw myself down a flight of stairs and, with luck, break my neck.

Good plan, right? Well, there were a couple of drawbacks. At that stage, I could still barely lift my arm up off the bed. I didn't have a motorized wheelchair yet. And even if I did, I wouldn't have been capable of getting myself into it and maneuvering it down the hall to the doors.

But I really didn't care about the drawbacks at that point. I had it all figured out. I was going to do it. Mentally, I just gave up, on therapy and everything else. Of course, they still made me go, so I was there physically. But I just didn't care. At best, it was a means of making me strong enough to lift myself into a chair, run it down the hall, ram the door, and fling myself down those stairs.

Kyla became my stand-in psychologist during my time in the dark spot. She and the other therapists knew about the divorce—I complained often enough—but of course there was nothing they could do about it. So, they stayed focused and kept pushing me forward. And while down there at MATC, I'd talk to Kyla about what was going on. I could be right in the middle of my mat, in one exercise or other, and start crying. I even told her that I wanted to kill myself. "No, John," she just said. "You can't do that. Because if you kill yourself, then you won't be my little playtoy and we won't be able to work together anymore." Like I mentioned, Kyla had a wicked sense of humor.

But my therapists were the only people I was emotionally letting in when I was down in the dark spot. As soon as I got back to my room, I would shut the door. I didn't want doctors in there; I didn't want nurses in there, either. No one. And they let me have my space. When my wife's mother was gone, I was finally, truly, on my own. Naturally, some of the mental health people at Walter Reed reached out to me. But I've hated psychologists since I was a kid, going through all that stuff with my mom. The staff tried their best to help me, but I wouldn't let them. Even if they forced their way into my room and started talking to me, I would just look at them with a blank, empty stare. My mind was made up. I was going to kill myself. I was just so ready to go, you know? *Fuck it, it's been a good life*, I thought to myself.

That's where I stayed, then, down in that dark spot, for maybe a month or two more.

Then one day, I was sitting in my room, looking out my fifth-floor window. And down below, I saw this wounded warrior. I didn't know who he was or the extent of his injuries, but I knew that he didn't have legs. He was sitting out in front of the hospital, and I could see he was wearing prosthetic legs. Maybe he was even a triple amputee, I didn't know. My first thought was *Oh, look, he's alone, too. We amputees are all going to be alone forever. Right now, he's probably thinking about crossing the street and throwing himself in front of a bus.* Well, suddenly, he got up, and he started walking toward the road. And I thought, *Yep, there he goes.* But the next thing I knew, a little girl ran up and grabbed his hand. He was looking down at her. He kept walking, and then a woman, who I assume was his wife, ran up, grabbed his waist, and the three of them walked off together.

Wait a second, I thought. *He's an amputee like me. He might have a limb or two more. But he's got someone holding onto him. Why can't I have that?* He got me thinking: *Maybe, just maybe, I should put the whole suicide plan on hold?*

One thing I did decide was to start talking to the staff again. And one of them was this Army licensed practical nurse named Michael Brown. As we're talking, he asked me if I've ever seen this TV show on the AMC network called *The Walking Dead,* about the world after a postzombie apocalypse. I had never seen it, but we started talking about zombies, and he told me that I would make a good one at Halloween with the right makeup. Halloween had just passed, I think, so that's why all this came up. Anyway, the second season of the show was about to start, and he said I really needed to see the first season before the new one began. I think my response was along the lines of "Whatever, dude, now get the hell out of my room." Even though I was talking to the staff, I was not bubbling over with friendliness.

Sure enough, the guy's back in my room the next day, asking me how my day is going and bringing along a DVD player. "You really need to watch this," he told me.

The Walking Dead is based on these graphic novels—okay, comic books— and the lead character is a deputy sheriff named Rick Grimes. He's shot in the line of duty and goes into a coma. When he finally wakes up, he's in a hospital, but he's all alone. No staff. No signs of life. The town outside the hospital walls is the same way. He's seemingly alone in this world overrun with zombies. He can't find his wife or son, or anyone else he knew from the way his life had been before. Eventually, he does find his family.

Now, I know this is fiction, but what it's about is this regular guy who is struggling, trying to find a way through these really dark times. And he puts it in his mind that he's going to do it. He's going to find his family. They are going to survive. "Maybe we got a second chance," Rick says during that first season. "Not many people get that."

As I watched the first episodes, I couldn't help but see similarities between his life, his struggle, and my own. I know it may sound a little corny, but you have to remember how down I was. Yes, I was making plans to kill myself, but somewhere there was this other part of me grasping at straws, looking for any way to get out of my own dark spot. So, between the wounded warrior I saw from my window and the story of Rick Grimes, I started thinking that maybe I wouldn't kill myself after all. Maybe it's not the best idea. There was no lightning bolt or anything like that. It was a slow but sure change of attitude.

For example, the next time I was in therapy, I made it a point to talk to Kyla. Not just about what a pain therapy is, or how it can seem pointless. And not about my ex-wife, either. Instead, I asked how her day was going. I asked how she was doing, how she was feeling. I asked what she did for fun when she wasn't messing around with her "little plank." I started doing the same on my hospital ward, trying to make some serious conversation with the nurses and the doctors. I think that was a bit of a shock to them. But I was determined to be a better man. To stop being so intense and angry. That wasn't me, and I wanted Kyla and the rest of staff to get to see that side of me that was living in the dark spot for far too long.

Many visitors come through Walter Reed. Some are family and loved ones of the wounded warriors, but a sizable number of celebrities and politicians like to visit, too. At one point during my dark spot, I heard some visitors going by my door, and I overheard one of the nurses or USO volunteers say to the person, "No, you don't want to go in there. He's not in the best place right now." Even my friend Gary Sinise remembers how angry I was and how tough it was for him to have a conversation with me. In fact, he mentioned that to me recently, and that came as no surprise, since I wasn't really social to so many people who were just trying to help. But you have to realize that such traumatic injuries carry with them unexpected consequences. Not only are you facing the reality that you might never walk again or feed yourself, but your mind is in the darkest place it has ever been. And I didn't want to be there anymore. That got me thinking too, believe me. So, for me to start being friendly with the staff, asking how their day was going, how their families were, that was a tremendous change; it was a shocker both for them and for me.

When you're on your own, recovering in a place like Walter Reed, you're constantly surrounded by people. But you can spend an awful lot of time alone, too. You can get stuck inside your own head. That's a killer. You sit, and you think. For quite a while, it was just me and my worst thoughts and my dark spot.

It scares me now to think about how close I came to giving in to that dark spot. I've overcome a lot of bad things in my life. But this, being a quad, was beyond any challenge I had ever imagined. Remember, I told Doc Gould to shoot me if I ever got this way.

What would my future be? After two soured marriages, would I ever find love again? I was worried about being alone, about being a drag on others. I was worried about the long, hard road to independence, or if I could even get there.

Then one day, I overheard one of the nurses say something that truly scared me. "You know," she said to another nurse outside my room, "I think we might need to send John to a nursing home."

THIRTEEN

BECOMING INDEPENDENT: NO NURSING HOME FOR ME

THAT CUT ME TO THE BONE. THERE I WAS, LYING IN A HOSPITAL BED WITH no arms or legs, wondering what my future would hold as a quadruple amputee. Then I heard those chilling words from one of the hospital administrators. "John, we don't think you can function independently anymore, so we would highly recommend that you consider going to a nursing home." A freakin' nursing home. *Are you fuckin' kidding?*, I thought, as she went on about what that would entail. I had to tune her out. "Hey, there is no way you're going to send me there," I said, as she looked at me, I guess trying to show some empathy. I told her in the strongest way possible: "Listen, I'm not helpless. I know I'm going to be independent someday, and I'm telling you right now that you better not send me to a nursing home."

But the truth is, I wasn't 100 percent sure of my capabilities. Unless you've been there, it's almost impossible to predict how you will heal. How long it will take for this part and that part to function again? I'm not going to lie. This time in my life was the absolute worst. The dark spot never fully went away. And now, all I could think of was getting out of it.

When I think back about the first blast, compared to the one in Afghanistan, it was a cake walk. I mean, losing your memory is no joke, but losing all four of your limbs is something that I wouldn't wish on anyone. The one good thing I learned after the first blast was the importance of perseverance, and never giving up. After the first blast, I learned I had to write every little thing down, with the clear goal of going back to my platoon and being a Marine again. I was determined not to let the memory issue affect the outcome of my life, and it didn't. So, based on that and my sheer willpower, I always believed that I could overcome anything. But when you don't have any arms or legs, can't hold a cup of coffee, touch your wife, or make a plate of scrambled eggs—man, that is totally different. (Of course, in truth, I had a wife in name only.)

Don't get me wrong. I had plenty of help from Kyla, my doctors, and some of the nurses, too. That evil administrator stopped by a couple more times, though she wasn't as much of a pain about the nursing home situation.

But that fear of becoming an invalid made me work even harder to get out of the hospital. There was no freakin' way I would ever end up in a nursing home. Period!

I was going through an hour of therapy every day. Finally, they got me an electric wheelchair, but to drive it, someone had to come with me to the MATC because they were concerned that I was having suicidal thoughts. Betty really did a number on me, that's for sure. And getting me in the chair was no easy task. I had to put the end of my left arm on the joystick to make it move. But I didn't have enough strength to push the joystick or even push the elevator buttons.

I also needed help out of bed and onto the wheelchair. They would lift me up with a bed sheet. It was awful. But I made a friend in the hospital, Bobby O'Neil, who was an Army specialist and one of my nurses. He was also a rabid Pittsburgh Steelers fan. I was a huge New England Patriots fan, and that became the beginning of a bet we made as we got to know each other better.

O'Neil wasn't the biggest guy in the world, but he was as strong as a bull. He wore a bright orange shirt, so I could see him coming a mile away. He would lift me up from the bed, bear-hug me, and literally toss me in the chair. It was extremely uncomfortable, especially since my skin was still very sensitive to the touch. But as my skin got better, O'Neil would just pick me up and throw me in the chair.

Once I got down to the MATC, Kyla was working on stretching my arms. Sgt. Webb, my occupational therapist, worked on my legs. Basically, they were both stretching me out little by little. As I got stronger, they would use bolsters, which are long, round pillows, but solid. They would put my right leg on the bolster and lift my butt off the ground. The purpose was to get me used to putting on prosthetics as well as getting as strong as possible. When I was done with my sessions, I would go back to my room, close the door, and sit and look out the window or watch my favorite Food Network shows or *Law and Order SVU*. Believe it or not, I still hadn't taken a shower for three months. The nurses would only give me bed showers. Kyla would joke around with me and ask me weird things like "Do you always do your hair?" She was referring to what looked like a cool spiked hairstyle but was really spiked because of three months of crud in my hair. "Good Lord, all that Afghan sand and dirt," she'd complain.

I guess the word was spreading that I needed to take a real shower, and I couldn't agree more. They actually had to make a plan for giving me my first shower, that's how nuts it was.

O'Neil was the chosen one, and he literally had to gown up in a special yellow gown, gloves, and booties. The next thing I knew, O'Neil picked me up with his bear hug and plopped me on the bench in the bathroom. He turned the water on, and the water immediately turned a brackish color from all the dirt. Totally disgusting! He washed my hair especially hard to get out all the soot, grime, and oil. I was shocked to see that a lot of my hair came out, too. It was literally dead hair. We did the shower thing only once, and then I noticed I was having pain in my ear; it turned out that I had a perforated eardrum. So, now I had to have another surgery on my right ear. The surgeons cut the back of my ear and folded it over, then took a piece of skin to make an eardrum. I must say, military medicine is awesome. I healed pretty quickly from that surgery, which was great.

There was another nurse I liked a lot. Her name was Elizabeth, and we had some great talks. One time when she was there, I ordered all this food—mozzarella sticks, tomato soup, and whatnot. Suddenly, I started vomiting bile—all this black stuff. Thankfully, Elizabeth was there.

Sometimes the assaults on my already broken body seemed endless. My balance was shitty. And it turned out after an optometry appointment they found out I had Afghan sand in my eye; sometimes we Marines refer to it as the "Afghan Funk." Luckily, it cleared up after only a few months.

I was still on methadone, a stool softener, and a blood thinner. Since my beard was growing in, and you know the Marines are not fond of facial hair, the nurses devised a plan. When I was medically sedated, they came into my room and gave me a proper shave. When I was more alert, I looked in the mirror and, to my horror, I had mutton chops. The nurses made me look like Elvis, of all things. I just cracked up. At times like this, I had to rely on my sense of humor to cope with the grim reality that I was a quadruple amputee.

But that was nothing compared to the gut punch I got soon afterward. As I was just starting to get back to myself, the Ward 58 Army administrator decided to stop by again for what I thought was just a friendly chat. "John," she said, "You don't have anybody—no wife, no mom, and there is no option for you. Plus, you can't stay at Walter Reed for the long term." Great news, huh? I asked O'Neil if he could be my caregiver, but he was on active duty and couldn't do it. Now we began having weekly meetings about what they were going to do with me.

But O'Neil was a funny and caring guy, and he knew just what to say and do to make me less of a pain in the ass. For example, one day he came into my room and had an interesting proposition.

"Let's make a bet," O'Neil said. "What is it?" I replied. "Okay, John, if Pittsburgh wins, you have to wear a Steelers jersey, and I'll wear the Pats jersey if New England wins, okay with you?" "That's fine," I said, "But if the Pats win, you have to shave my pubic hair in the shower." He agreed. Of course, the Pats won. Enough said! O'Neil was a great friend, and he helped me not be such a dick, and for that I'm forever grateful. I never saw him much after that time because he went on deployment.

Despite my physical and emotional improvement, the nursing home option was still on the table after I was discharged. I thought, "Wait, hold on, you're going to send a guy who's already suicidal to an old person's place to die? I'm not going to have any friends there. Seriously? Okay, you're trying to get rid of me, right?"

But they didn't seem to take me seriously. Still, I was determined to get myself stronger, become more independent, and show them that a nursing home was not a viable alternative.

So, I was working harder than ever on my OT and PT. I was beginning to get my sense of humor back, too. So, one day, O'Neil and this blonde Army captain came into my room, and I asked her, "Are you single?" She told me "No, I'm not." She told me that her fiancé, an Army doctor, also worked at Walter Reed. I took a look at her ring finger and saw her engagement ring. Don't ask me why I said this, but I said, "If you dump him, I'll get you an even bigger engagement ring." I was pulling on her chain, of course.

Another example was that sometimes, when it was time for my meds, I would get in my chair and yell to the nurses, "Ha-ha, you can't catch me," and they would proceed to chase me around the ward. At least I thought it was funny. Another time, I took one of the lab coats that I somehow got my hands on. Someone helped put the jacket on me, and I proceeded to visit the OBGYN ward just down the hallway. I went into one of the exam rooms and said with as earnest an expression as I could muster, "Hi, my name is Dr. Peck, and I'm here to do your examination." They all cracked up. Clearly, I was feeling a lot better.

I also made a few friends who were fellow patients, like this master sergeant who jumped out of a C130, hit his head on the plane, and broke his neck. He came to Walter Reed right around the time I did, and his room was next to mine. He had a girlfriend. She apparently asked about me and was wondering if I had any regular visitors. I guess she heard I was all alone. One morning, she came to my room and stood next to my bed and said, "Hi, I'm Julie, and I wanted to stop by and see how you're doing." I looked at her with my head tilted since I still couldn't turn my body. "Who are you?" I asked. "And how old are you and are you single?" She cracked up and said she wasn't. She was nice to visit me, and she obviously recognized that I needed some cheering up.

It was around this time they decided I needed to be fitted for prosthetic legs. To make a fit for my right leg, I had to have a casting made. So, I had to get buck naked in front of this dude named Mike. He was six feet five and from Ireland. To begin this process, Mike said this: "All right, John, I'm going to get you naked now." *Well, that sounds like fun,* I thought. To do the casting properly, I had to put on these little cloth shorts. I thought, *No way, they're way too short and tight.* But in truth, my skin was getting better to touch, and hey, you gotta do what you gotta do.

But that embarrassment was nothing compared to what came next.

One day, I decided to call Betty, just to check in and let her know about my progress. I knew that things were really bad between us, but to be honest, the last thing I needed at this point was to have to deal with relationship problems, let alone go through another divorce. "Hey, Betty, I got great news today. I stood on my leg for the very first time." And this is what she said to me—verbatim: "Why the fuck do you think I care? I don't give a fuck, why don't you kill yourself now and make the world a better place. No woman's ever going to love you anyway."

Those were horrible, evil words. They cut me to the bone. By mid-November, I started to make the decision to officially get a divorce. I asked Betty, "How can you be so cruel, what was going on with you?" She basically said she was going through stuff herself, and the loss of my limbs affected her psychologically. No shit! What did *she* think *I* was going through? I was happy before I talked to her, then afterward I was crushed. Plus, I was by myself. Someone asked me how I was going to deal with it. I had no idea, and the question put me right back in the dark spot again. I was alone. Not loved by a woman. I would die here alone. But, as usual, I found a reason to pull myself out of it. I realized that I could still enrich my life with friends and what family I had left.

When I thought about the other quads like me, I realized they had people who loved them. Brandon had his dad and brother, and Todd had his wife. Then there was me. I had to believe I would find someone, even as a quad.

I told everybody, "You know I understand, but here's the one thing. You guys have wives and family, but I'm alone plus going through a monstrous divorce. The injury was bad enough. Screw the injury, it's the divorce I can't handle."

The divorce was as messy as a divorce can be in terms of the typical stuff—dividing income and all of that. I had to make sure Betty didn't take any more of my money or possessions, but I had the added annoyance of having to deal with lawyers and legal fees. I guess very few people are fortunate enough to have amicable divorces. But what made it really hurt was Betty's verbal abuse and lack of empathy. I'm sure I'm way more sensitive to the verbal abuse than most—I had enough of that for two lifetimes. In addition, I hate failure of any kind, and having yet another divorce on my record was something I hated. No matter how Betty explained her behavior to me and why she did what she did, still, it was a bitter pill to swallow. How could someone be so cruel and heartless to another human being? While I had my share of abuse and rejection before—thank you, Mike and Adam—what Betty did was even more stinging. Loyalty is very important to me. I wouldn't leave my buddies behind no matter what. And I would never have abandoned Betty if she were in the same situation. That's just me. But fortunately, a great new development at the hospital helped take my mind off it. I got my first prosthetic arm, called a myoelectric arm. I was beginning to feel whole again. It attached to my missing right elbow, and on the right side were the controls. I unbended my elbow, basically pushing my right arm down, pulling the string to unlock the elbow. The goal was to make my back smaller and wingspan bigger. On the right side was a loop that ran on my back to my left arm. Sensors inside the socket lined up with my biceps and triceps. The switch for the wrist was easy to adjust with sensors, depending on how weak or strong I was at the time. I had someone helping me with my lower prosthetic and another person with my upper prosthetic.

For those who know nothing about these high-tech devices, prosthetics have made great strides over the years since they have been in use—even as far back as 1600, if you can believe it. After the Second World War, with so many warriors missing limbs, the military began to conduct research to develop prosthetic devices. Today, they have been greatly improved through robotics and other innovations. I'm sure someday, they will even be able to regenerate a person's missing limbs. But for now, I would be only one of five quadruple amputees from the War on Terror to have to be fitted for not just one or two—but four prosthetic limbs. Lucky me!

For the hand, they gave me what is called a "Greifer," a powerful, highly functional mechanical hand. It can literally crush a damn can. It works extremely well—maybe too well. That was evident when one of the therapists walked out of the room for a second, and I was just sitting there scratching my nose and the damn thing opened! It was a big hook, and it started to close on my nose. Forty pounds of pressure per square inch. Shit, that hurt. It was very painful, and when the therapist came back and saw what had happened, he was really upset. "Oh my God, dude, I'm sorry." "I'm okay, but it hurts," I replied. That was a trip. For my left arm, things went a little smoother. I had a powered prosthetic to help with the damaged biceps. This device helped my arm bend. It was the same concept that if I pushed the left arm down, it would lock or unlock my elbow.

I was a walking, talking transformer.

But despite my progress in getting used to my new prosthetics, it was a struggle for me. What were once two strong arms that were able to perform complicated tasks were now mechanical contraptions. My legs that carried me through war zones in Iraq and Afghanistan were now nothing more than stubs—with one cut so high that it was almost impossible to fit a prosthetic leg. I would be lying if I said that I had faith that I would become whole again. As I said before, prosthetic legs did not really work for me.

And, at this point in my recovery, I still had no idea where or when I would be leaving the hospital. One day during therapy, Kyla and I were talking, and I told her about the nursing home. She asked me, "John, have you thought about reconnecting with your mom?" I said that that was a great idea, and so the next day I asked someone to help me dial the phone.

It was the call that kept me from the worst of fates—a nursing home.

My mom and I had a good conversation, and we ended up talking quite a few times. During one of the calls, I said to my mom, "I'm sorry about what happened, and I'm sorry I believed the lies about you that Betty kept telling me. Hey, do you think you could come here to help me?" She replied, "Absolutely." I was relieved.

During the next few weeks, we had more meetings with the administrator and others, and I told them that my mom was willing to take care of me. They said, "Wow, your mom can't come back." I asked, "Why not?" They said, "John, your mom was forbidden from coming here, and she was escorted out."

"Guys, it was me," I said. "I'm the one who initiated that, and since I did then, now I'm saying it's okay for her to come back." They took my word but as always had another plan for my future. They requested both my mom and I take a psych exam. Then we had to sit down with the Marine liaison. Before I brought my mom back, my grandparents were an option, as well. But my grandfather said he couldn't come without my grandmother, and she would have to get paid, too. "John, if I come, my wife has to come with me, and we need to figure out what we're going to do with our two dogs," my grandfather told me. "Well, you can't bring them to Walter Reed," I told him, because of the hospital's strict rules. "John, I'm sorry, but I can't get rid of our dogs." I said, "Are you serious? I came to your house all the time and mowed your lawn and fixed stuff. You mean to tell me that you would choose your dogs over your grandson?" I was crushed.

On the positive side, I now had my mom on her way and keeping me from that dreaded nursing home.

But before she arrived, something great happened. There was a Marine down the hall who was a single amputee. He had a sister. His mom was there, too, and they wanted to talk to anyone who didn't have all their family with them. The next thing I knew, his sister came into my room on New Year's Eve. I was sound asleep, of course. She woke me up just before midnight and kissed me on the cheek. *What's going on?* I thought. I realized I was still married, but I was in the process of a divorce, so what the hell. That kiss felt wonderful. She was twenty-five and in college, and one thing led to another.

We dated for a few months. But soon we broke up because her family got in the way. They didn't want her to leave school and help me as a caregiver. I did understand and was thankful for the intimate experience. But rumors started to fly. People said they heard me and my major talking in the hallway, and I told him she gives great blow jobs. I have never had a conversation in my life like that. Really? Come on!

I really liked this girl. It wasn't like I thought, *Oh my God, she's awesome.* But she gave me the boost I needed, and it got me back on track again. Some people have asked me how I coped with all of this. I'm not sure, to be honest. It's just something I do. It's just how I handle things; I can't break it down. I guess I'm biologically built that way, and my brain handles information as methodically as a computer.

My mom came to stay with me in February 2011. We moved to the Malone House at the old Walter Reed. The Malone House provides families of wounded warriors being treated at Walter Reed a home away from home. The VA also pays wounded warrior caregivers, which made it possible for her to give up her job to come and be with me. We had two queen beds, but hardly enough room to pull my chair in. We even had to take the bathroom door off, just so that I could get around. It was almost like a college dorm setup. But even though I was getting my life together, my nightmare with Betty wasn't over.

As it turns out, divorced Marines have to pay half of their salary to their ex-wives. Since I didn't want to mess up because of my disability, I set up an auto-pay service at the bank. But because sometimes the auto-pay day fell on a weekend, then the payment was delayed a day or two. When that occasionally happened, Betty would call the command and tell them that she wasn't paid. At the time, I received $2,400 a month and her cut was $1,200. Since it was on auto-pay, there was no way she didn't get the money.

But despite all the shit I was going through with Betty, I was still working hard on my PT and OT. Tyler Southern and I would work out on an upstairs track that went around the gym. They had a climbing wall on the lower level. While we were doing our OT, the people downstairs told us that we were still Marines and had to follow the policy at the gym to wear black shorts and ugly green shirts. Since we had no control over our body heat because our limbs were gone, those shorts and shirts made us sweat beyond belief. (That's because our blood does not have enough room to travel before it goes back to the heart. As blood travels down the extremities and back, it cools, but for us that didn't happen. Our bodies always feel blistering hot.) They also warned us that facial hair was a no-no; but, seriously, it's really tough to shave when you don't have any arms.

Then we got a new captain named Capt. Henderson. He walked past me when I was doing my therapy and gave me a real hard look. Then he took a few steps back and said to me, "Cpl. Peck." I replied, "Yes sir." "Can I ask you a question? What do you think about shaving your face?" *Are you serious,* I thought? "Well, sir, when my arms grow back, I can shave." He gave me a look. "I'm serious, corporal, when are you going to shave your face?" I couldn't help myself at this point. "Sir, when I get done with more important things like therapy, so I can use my prosthetic arm to pick up a razor, I'll shave my face. Plus, you can ask my mother, and she'll confirm that I'm on blood thinners, and if I cut myself with a razor, that could spell big trouble." He wasn't impressed. "Who is your squad leader?" he asked me.

I had to tell him, of course. Later that day, my squad leader came into my room and said, "Cpl. Peck, what the hell did you say to the new captain?" No kidding, I thought the entire incident was hilarious. I told my squad leader, SSGT Ramirez, that I wasn't trying to be a dick about it. You have to remember that I was just getting over an injury. It took me forty-five minutes just to get ready in the morning, and I was only sleeping about three or four hours a night. I explained to him that every small task that I would do quickly before the blast literally took three or four times longer than it did before. For example, someone would have to help me get out of bed, put me in a wheelchair, roll it into the shower, and help me wash up. Then they would dry me off, brush my teeth, comb my hair, and do all those basic hygiene things that guys do. Then came the challenge of getting me dressed, putting me back in the chair, feeding me breakfast, and then finally helping me leave the apartment. It was completely exhausting.

In addition, we amputees experience what they call phantom pain. They call it "phantom" because our brains still experience pain in the limbs that we lost. So, I would actually feel pain in my arms and legs—sometimes excruciating—even though I don't have any. It's quite a surreal experience.

The other thing that happened—once my mom had been back for a few months—was another Betty gut punch, a big one. I wasn't in the dark spot anymore, but still this one really hurt.

After my mom and I were at the Malone House for a bit, I called Betty to ask about Diesel, my Shiba Inu. "Betty, I need my stuff and I want to get Diesel back." She said with zero emotion, "Well, I gave Diesel to our neighbor. Then, Diesel pooped on his carpet and he punished him, and Diesel bit him." I knew this was bullshit. Diesel was gentle and was just defending himself from abuse, like I had to do as a kid. Anyway, they quarantined him, but he didn't have rabies.

Then Betty gave me even worse news. "John, we had to put Diesel down." I was so sad and pissed off at the same time. I could hardly speak. I managed to say, "Hey, can you at least get my stuff from the apartment, especially my uniform and 350z." She went silent; I hung up the phone.

I was so depressed but finally decided to ask some of my friends from California if they wouldn't mind going to the apartment and retrieving my things. I wish Diesel could have been part of that. When they got there, they found all my uniforms were torn up, all my medals ripped, and someone even urinated on my uniform. My car was also damaged. I immediately called Betty. "What the hell did you do to my uniform?" "John, it wasn't me. Some homeless guy broke in," she said. She was lying. "Bullshit, Betty, you did that same shit to your ex-husband," I said. "You and your friend destroyed his uniforms, too. Your crazy friend even put a toothbrush in her butt and rubbed it on his stuff. And it's a load of crap to tell me a homeless person broke in. Do you think I'm stupid?"

It was another bad trip down memory lane. This divorce couldn't come soon enough. But as luck would have it, some of my friends from Antioch and some guys from my unit stepped up to the plate to help me. They not only sent me my stuff, but they found out I owed $1,000 on my rent. They paid the entire bill, no questions asked; I would have done the same thing for them.

But when they were actually in my car, they found it was filled with Afghan sand. In the meantime, our congressman from Illinois learned about my situation and wanted to meet me. When he learned what happened to my car, he called me and said, "John, don't worry; I got it." Gene, who was going to drive the car back for me, took it to an auto dealer. They repaired the damage free of charge, thanks to the congressman. At the same time, some military recruiters from Chicago found out about my situation and performed a true act of kindness. It was something I will never forget.

Believe it or not, they drove from Chicago to Walter Reed and plotted an unusual course. They brought a Marine Corps flag with them, then stopped at every recruiter along the way. Each time, the recruiter signed the flag, and many wrote kind messages. When they finally arrived at the hospital, it was filled with signatures. I was moved. In fact, so much so that I hung it behind the door in my room. Did I mention they also gave me an NCO sword that I kept in a scabbard? It even had a nice cloth bag. I was so proud of that flag. Unlike Vietnam veterans, today's wounded warriors enjoy tremendous public support. In fact, there are literally hundreds, if not thousands, of nonprofit organizations across the country that are dedicated to helping wounded warriors and their families in a host of ways. From very large groups like the USO to small, basically "mom and pop" shops, they really have made a difference. And the fact that my hometown was so supportive by giving me this symbol of freedom helped to lift my spirits and gave me a renewed sense of purpose, and added to my resolve to help others in need.

I had the flag framed. People would stop by to visit, including some generals, sergeant majors, and commandants. They signed my flag and also gave me their challenge coins. All my guys from Afghanistan signed a Marine Corps flag and sent it to me, as well. Even President Obama, who was winding down the troop commitment in Afghanistan by then, gave me his challenge coin, but it turned out that Betty kept it.

Another random act of kindness occurred when I was still an inpatient. Jim Hoover, who was a major with the Marines, saw my story. He was stationed in Quantico and decided to visit me. He heard I was a Pats fan. So, you know what he did? He contacted the NFL and asked them if he could get a game day Pats jersey signed for me by none other than quarterback Tom Brady. But they went a step further, and the entire team signed the jersey, except for Randy Moss. They even gave me the football that was used during the game. The Pats won that game by a field goal, by the way.

With everything I'd been through, my injury and impending divorce, I knew I could always count on my friends from my hometown of Antioch. I decided to come home for a few days to personally tell them how much I appreciated their support. We did this in May of 2011, partly so I could celebrate my "alive day" of May 24 with them. (Injured warriors call this the day we were injured but survived.)

My mom and I drove back to Illinois, and apparently a foundation found out about what happened to my dog Diesel. My mom put together a blood drive to replenish the blood supply I used during my treatments. It was held at our local VFW. A few days later, and to my surprise, a group of older women told me to pick out any dog I wanted from our local pet store.

These caring, Midwestern, down-to-earth folks gave me hope that the world was in fact a good place and let me know I wasn't alone. It was so awesome to see all our little town's residents lined up shoulder to shoulder along Main Street to wave to me as I drove by. I felt tears well up in my eyes, but good Marine that I was, I tried to hold them back.

Once we got settled, my mom and I went to the pet store and found my dog. She was a purebred husky. Straight up, she could see through your soul with her intense blue eyes. She had beautiful black, white, and gray markings, and I named her Misha. I put her in my lap and she kept licking me; dogs are my soft spot.

Sadly, my mom and I weren't the only ones who were affected by my memory loss. Some of the folks in Antioch were shocked to realize I had no idea who they were. This one guy I went to school with came up to me and said: "Hey John, we went to school together, don't you remember me?"

"Man, I'm sorry," I said, "but I don't know who you are."

Seeing my old friends and not having a clue who they were made me feel awful. But I was lucky to have my mom working with me to help me remember things. She tried to jog my memory by showing me scrapbooks, family pictures, and she talked to me constantly to help me remember who I was and where I came from. And it's funny. Despite not really remembering who they were, it was somehow comforting to see my old friends and to try to remember who they were.

I took Misha with me to an event with my old high school friend, Kymmie, who had a disease of the spine and had to walk on crutches. "Do you remember me?" said Kymmie. "You should, John, because you stood up for me so many times in high school." *Why can't I remember this one?,* I thought. "People were always bullying me, and you were right there," Kymmie said. I was touched.

I would take Misha over to see Kymmie, and we would catch a smoke. I felt I was home again.

But when we got back to Walter Reed, I encountered some new problems. This one lady who was also injured caused a ruckus for me. She told me, "You can't have a dog here." I said, "Hey, I got it cleared." Then she said, and I was completely thrown off by this, "Please understand I'm injured, as you can see. You think I was born this ugly?"

What the hell? "I don't know if you were ugly, come on," I said. "I just found out my wife gave my dog away, then killed the dog. I'm injured, and I could use the support of my new dog." She didn't seem to get it. Also, that nasty captain who gave me a hard time about shaving repeated his mean behavior. "Cpl. Peck, you need to get rid of the dog, and you need to do it by Saturday." So, after about a month, we were forced to go back to Illinois, where I had to give Misha to Gene.

But despite all the bullshit I went through, I knew deep down that I wouldn't be this way forever. Sure, I was a quadruple amputee, but I had to leave the dark spot behind. This was another one of those times when I needed to compartmentalize my pain, deal with whatever challenge comes my way, and move on. So I did.

Then I remembered another bright spot. When I was an inpatient, Frank Siller and John Ponte, from Tunnel to Towers, a nonprofit organization that builds homes for severely injured wounded warriors, came into my room and said that when I was better, they would be honored to build a custom smart home for me. That was the beginning of my independence, emotional stability, and the motivation to move on. Despite all I had to deal with—especially the hurt I felt when Betty abandoned me and spewed such venom—I wouldn't change a thing. In fact, if any one of the small details in my life changed from what they were, those changes might have prevented me from being who I am and where I am today. I'm a firm believer that you should never look back but always be happy where you are at the moment. Call it my survival gene.

FOURTEEN

BETHESDA BOUND:
MY RECOVERY CONTINUES

IN AUGUST 2011, I WAS TRANSFERRED TO THE NEW WALTER REED NATIONAL Military Medical Center, which had just opened. I didn't have a van at that time, so my mom and I were a little worried about how we would get all our stuff over to Bethesda, not to mention me and my wheelchair. And being transferred to Bethesda would mean I would be an outpatient and continue my PT and OT, but in much nicer surroundings. Unlike the old Walter Reed, there would be no mice or ceiling leaks.

Some of my therapists would continue with me in Bethesda, but Kyla wasn't one of them. That made me sad, because Kyla was the one person who could make me laugh, listen to me when I was down and out, and help me recognize that I was still a person worthy of love and respect—despite being a quad. Unfortunately, she would be transferred, and a woman named Kerry would be my new physical therapist. Before we moved, I teased Kyla, telling her, "Kyla, you dropped me as a patient." She cracked up. She was a champ!

My mom and I had accumulated a lot of stuff, and we were wondering what to do with it during the move. That's when the nonprofit Semper Fi Fund, which I really like, stepped up by renting us an adapted van. Our new apartment at Bethesda was actually pretty nice. It was in Building 62, which you may remember as the place where wounded warriors stay after they become outpatients.

We had a small living room, kitchen, and two separate bedrooms, each with their own bathroom. My mom and I were living in very close quarters, and there were times when we fought a lot. Sometimes over stupid things like me yelling at her for hovering around me like I was a total invalid. It just happens. Living in such tight quarters would make anyone crazy. Plus, I needed constant attention and care, so she sometimes neglected her own needs. I'm sure she still had some anger toward me for asking her to leave the hospital after the second blast, but then my mom knew me all too well and understood that too would pass. Despite the issues we always had with each other, she was still my mom, and I was her son. Those bonds, though often challenged, always remained strong. To help us deal with our issues, my mom and I went to see a psychiatrist to get some help living together in peace. I'm happy to report that counseling really helped us. Our fights were not as bad, and having her there was actually comforting to me.

I also started to make friends with guys like Adam Keys, Clark Cavalier, Tyler Southern, and Mike Frazier. They were all wounded warriors, most with amputations and other medical problems; we are friends to this day. They totally got it, and we had one another's backs. But there were some other amputees at Bethesda who gave me a really hard time, if you can believe that.

I told you earlier about my problems with prosthetics. Still, I sometimes tried walking with my new prosthetic legs along the ramp of the complex. These were "shorty" legs, low to the ground to help you get more proficient at walking, so at some point you can be fitted for full-length prosthetics. But the pain, especially in my left leg, was excruciating. It was just easier to get around in my wheelchair. One day, I was walking on my shorties, and one of the quads with a set of new prosthetic knees passed me and said, "Hey Mr. Peck," and he knew that pissed me off because we rarely use ranks and titles to address one another, "Why don't you have your prosthetic knees? I've only been injured six months, and I already have my prosthetic knees." What a heartless thing to say to a fellow quad. I don't remember exactly what I said to him, but I pointed out that he was married and had a lot more support than I had at the time. I've always tried to encourage others to be their personal best. We all think and heal differently, and any guy who has been injured serving his country in any way should be treated with empathy and respect. This guy clearly didn't get it. Plus, while he was another quad, we had very different amputations. He had a left residual leg, whereas I had absolutely nothing. That made walking on prosthetics 200 percent more difficult for me.

The truth was that my injury was complicated, like that of some of my other buddies. Like I said before, it's hard for me to use prosthetic legs when one leg is disarticulated at the hip. There's literally nothing to attach to a prosthetic leg. Plus, the artificial legs are very heavy, and even if I did have the perfect stumps, there would still be discomfort and pain. And even though I was getting more proficiency with my prosthetic arms, I still wasn't anywhere near independent. I needed help with basic things like pouring water, eating, and taking a shower. That's because my new arms did not have the ability to perform the fine motor tasks, and they were almost impossible to use when I needed to lift them up above my head to do a simple thing like comb my hair. While people who see us guys on TV think our prosthetics are a piece of cake, I can tell you they're not.

I had so many insecurities to overcome. After all, look at me. I'm not physically who I was before. But over time, I was beginning to feel more confident, compared to when I was first blown up. But, honestly, I did have my doubts about whether anyone would ever be attracted to me again. Betty's cruel words echoed in my mind. I had to overcome them by sheer will, tenacity, and the determination to get back to who I was before my injury. I had to summon my inner strength.

One of the ways I found that strength was with my new friends, and we took some trips to the beach in the summer, thanks to a nonprofit called Waterfront Warriors. They were awesome. One of their volunteers was this big New York firefighter. He would lift me up, put me in a beach chair, and even rub suntan lotion all over me, which was weird but necessary. This one girl was helping out at the waterfront camp who I thought was cute. She came up to me on the beach and said, "Hey, you know I can get you a pizza if you want." I guess either I didn't hear her, or I was consumed by my thoughts. She walked away but came back later. "Hey, Mr. Grumpy."

"Are you talking to me?" I replied.

"Yeah, I was talking to you and why didn't you answer me?" I told her that I didn't hear her and that I was sorry. "Hey, I'll take that pizza," I said to her. After that, she gave me her number, surprising me with her overture. I sent her a text message. It read: "Hey, I'm staying at a nice hotel. Do you want to come over and hang out?" One thing led to another, and we began dating. That lasted for quite a few months, and she even came to visit me multiple times. She lived in Staten Island, New York, but she moved down to Virginia after she got her college degree to be close to me. It was fun while it lasted, but we broke up six months later. But having this brief but very satisfying relationship gave me the jolt of confidence I needed to feel whole again. I have to admit that I was insecure with women. Hey, who wouldn't be if they suddenly went from a self-proclaimed stud to a quadruple amputee?

Meanwhile, that summer, my divorce from Betty was lingering on and becoming even more troublesome. As I mentioned earlier, the people from my hometown hosted a number of fundraisers to help me. They hosted a car show, sold t-shirts, and staged other events to raise money. After a few months, they sent me a check for $56,000. But when Betty left for California, never to return, she took the check with her. Then she tried to cash it a few days later. When I went to the bank to take out some money a day or two later, not knowing what Betty did, Ramirez and I both heard the bank teller say, "Sir, there aren't enough funds in your account, and it looks like someone in California was trying to cash your check." I called the bank in Antioch and put a stop payment order on the check. Then they reissued a new check directly to me. As you can imagine, after this, I really stepped up my divorce proceedings. I was done! I should have done this much earlier, but I was more focused on my recovery than having to deal with all of the crap of a divorce. There were obviously serious financial negotiations, as well as jurisdiction issues. I was hopeful that soon this nightmare would be over.

And it was. We were married on Valentine's Day, and our divorce was final in October 2011. It was just a regular, normal day, but to me it was a holiday and time for a real celebration!

Free of Betty, I was on a good track, both mentally and physically. That's when I decided to bring some of my friends together and figure out a way to do something good for someone else. I'd read that helping others can improve your outlook on life. As you know by now, when I was growing up, we only had the basics. And being raised by a working single mother, I knew how tough the holidays were. When the other kids would get the gift they asked for, I would just get a pair of socks. Let me tell you, Christmas sucks for the poor. That's when I got the idea I was going to help people in need during the holidays, especially single mothers. That's an idea, as you'll see later, that I've put into practice a lot.

Also, at Bethesda, I asked my staff sergeant if I could put something together on each ward for the inpatient Marines. He liked the idea and gave me a list of all the injured Marines in the hospital. I would describe it as a peer-to-peer visitation program. I wanted all Marines to have another Marine visit them. I know how much it helped me when I was in the hospital to be able to talk to someone who understood my situation. The peer-to-peer program worked really well, but after a while, my own physical and occupational therapy took more and more of my time, and the program went by the wayside. I couldn't oversee it like I had wanted, but I was proud that I made the effort to focus on something other than myself. That was one of the important life lessons I learned from my mom—the responsibility we all have to give back to our fellow man. To be a helper, not a parasite.

Besides, all of us amputees had plenty of other visitors when we were in-patient and even when we were rehabilitating. Honestly, many of us thought that some of the celebrities who came to our rooms were more interested in photo-ops—their own publicity—than spending time with us. It really pissed me off when they would all be so sickeningly nice. They would give us their cards and tell us we could call them anytime. But when we would try to contact them, there was no response. We got really good at spotting the bullshitters. They're the ones who think they are so great just because they act in a movie or sing. Really? But don't get me wrong, there were others who were genuine and awesome.

Gary Sinise was one of them. I know how committed he is to helping wounded warriors and veterans as well as first responders. Hey, he and Tunnel to Towers would eventually build my smart home, and Gary's band—the Lt. Dan Band, from his role in *Forrest Gump*—would host a fundraising concert for me to help pay for it. And I was surprised to learn that one of Gary's good pals, the actor and director Clint Eastwood, donated $100,000 of his own money to help pay for my home. He didn't want any publicity about the donation, which made me respect him even more.

Another one of the famous people I met back at the Malone House was Chef Carla Hall. Well, maybe she wasn't famous to everyone, but she sure was to me. I was stoked. We spent hours talking just about food; it was cool to meet somebody like her and be able to have such interesting conversations. I've also heard through the grapevine that celebrities like musician Roger Waters and Prince Harry were the real deal and to this day support wounded warriors. Prince Harry spends tons of time talking to warriors when he visits. He also created the "Invictus Games," where guys like me can compete in sports like archery.

After only about a few months in Bethesda, I was almost beginning to be able to feed myself with my new prosthetic arms. But it's not easy and, in fact, can be seriously dangerous, at least concerning food, as I found out one time in the Warrior Café. I was playing around in the cafeteria and accidentally stabbed a hush puppy with my arm. It was embarrassing, but the guys around me cracked up. After that, I had another idea to start a cooking group for all the amputees. Actually, it was a grilling group; Caitlin, my physical therapist, led it. I figured the guys with prosthetic arms could use them for skewers. Not!

The other thing that happened to me in Bethesda was following up with a guy I met at the Malone House. His name was Harvey Navarro. He thought that I should get a service dog, because he knew how the loss of my dogs, Misha and Diesel, affected me. I told Harvey that I would love to have a service dog. "Harvey, when I have a dog, I'm better and happier." Harvey recommended a few organizations, including Canine Companions for Independence, which is well regarded and provided service dogs for some of my friends.

I was accepted into their program, and soon a woman came to Bethesda with a kind of practice dog for me to meet. His name was Hercules. She said, "John, I don't know how we're going to attach a leash to you. But we'll figure it out before your class."

She taught me how to work with Hercules. I learned the basic commands, plus some that were unique to me. For example, I would put Hercules on the right side of my chair and tell him, "Let's go," so we were moving at the same time. The commands had to be very authoritative; none of that soft stuff. Hercules was a great dog, but they wanted to pair me up with the dog for my specific needs and personality. They also explained that training a service dog could take a while.

I was ready. It must have been only another month or so when I got a call from Canine Companions for Independence. They found a dog for me. Hooray!

They told us that we had to come to New York to meet the dog. But there was one catch. At the time, Bethesda didn't allow service dogs on the base. That isn't the case today. But back then, I knew how much a dog meant to me and the other wounded warriors, so I was compelled to act. I spoke to the commanding officer of the Marine Corps liaison at Bethesda and let him know I planned to appeal to my congressman. After some back-and-forth, the base commander apparently decided to allow service dogs on base. That was a good day.

As you'd expect, there were some new rules for service dogs on base. We had to get a note from a doctor, have proof that we graduated from the service dog training class, and a few other conditions. That was fine by me.

So, off we went. Mom and I drove to New York. We stayed at CCI's facility. We didn't have to pay a penny, and all the food was free. It was quite a learning experience. We couldn't meet our dog until we completed classes and learned all the commands, like sit, down, stay, and come, among others. After all that, they introduce you to the dogs. They try to match each dog with the right warrior, making sure the personality of the dog meets what the warriors need. I had to find a dog that had high energy yet could still chill. The first dog we met was too mellow. The second dog, named Nasar, was another story. He was two years old—a yellow Lab mixed with a golden retriever. Nasar was named for the National Association of Search and Rescue.

It was love at first sight. The first thing that Nasar did was hop on my lap then began smelling my arm. He was adorable. I knew he was the dog for me.

My mom soon brought her dog Bailey to New York to meet Nasar. Luckily, they hit off. About a week after we were matched with Nasar, I had him jump on the bed; I couldn't resist. But the rules still applied to Mom. She wasn't allowed to pet Nasar or pay attention to him. I had a learning curve, too, because at times I was being too commanding. There was a fine line, even for dogs, and sometimes my tone was too stern. But soon, Nasar and I were going on public outings at places like the Bass Pro Shop. The goal was for me to gain confidence in handling him. And I also learned that I had to let other people know that service dogs are not pets. They can't be touched or distracted. There are many more rules for service dogs, and that is important for the welfare of the warrior and the dog, as well.

My mom and I returned to Bethesda, with Nasar as part of the team.

After more months of therapy, I realized that the things I loved to do before my injury, like playing video games, I just couldn't do anymore. So, we decided to go to a hobby store to find something I could buy that would be fun and I could do with my prosthetic arms. We decided to buy a remote-control car. I had a hard time controlling the car with my Greifer and crashed the thing multiple times. One day when I was at occupational therapy, I mentioned my problem with the remote-control car to Caitlin. She said, "John, I have an idea. There is a guy who comes here and adapts all kinds of things, so they can enjoy what they used to before."

"That's cool," I said.

"His name is Ken Jones and he's an engineer from New Jersey. I'll let him know that you want something adapted."

A month later, Ken came down to meet me, and I showed him my remote-control car and the problem I was having with it. "Let me figure this out, John, I think I can come up with something for you." Three weeks later, he came back with a crazy contraption that took some getting used to. He attached a removable joystick to my chair that controlled my car. All I had to do was basically drive a wheelchair to work the car.

It worked like a charm. When I told Adam Keys about the car, he wanted one, too. So, when he bought his, we would go to the park on weekdays after our therapy and spend hours and hours playing with our new toys.

After Ken learned about the success of his contraption, he asked me if there was anything else I wanted to do. "Hey, thanks, Ken. The one thing I loved before I got injured was playing video games. Do you have any interest in figuring that out?" I asked.

"Yeah, John, you would be the first quad I've ever done, but I think I could make it work," Ken replied.

"Man, I'm not expecting anything," I said, "but thanks for trying to figure that out."

Ken would make the three-hour drive from New Jersey to Maryland many times to figure out how to make this work for me. Finally, he came back with the test model, basically a free-standing table-top base. To use it, I had to move my leg toward or away from my groin, and up so I could hit the controls. My right arm controls the right joystick, then my left arm moves the left joystick. So, there are three different switches. In the past, most of my video games were fast and complex, but my first game with my new device was not fast or high speed. We bought it at GameStop, and it was something like Star Wars or Lego Batman. But that simple, easy, and slow game gave me something I lost; I was grateful. It took a lot of work for Ken to create both my devices, but he didn't stop there.

Since I was a smoker, which I'm not anymore, it took a lot of work to light a cigarette. I just couldn't do it. Ken decided he could fix that problem, too. He took an old school lighter from a car and ran a current through the coil. So, to smoke, all I had to do was press a button, and it would light my cigarette. Ken also designed a paintball gun with a motorized turret attached to my chair with little holes for attachments. The paintball gun was mounted, and the joystick was for my right hand and the button for my left arm. Ken is one person I throw my name behind. He did all this work for free, and it was just him and one other guy.

I think the cost for the paintball adaptations was around $750; Ken paid for each one. Ken's organization called "Warfighters Engaged" does not take donations from wounded warriors. But one time, I gave him $1,000 and told him he had to keep the money. He was touched. "John, without donations like yours, we couldn't do all the things to keep you and your warfighters engaged. I didn't want to accept your check, but I know how serious you are about supporting what we do," Ken said. I could never repay him for what he gave back to me. Ken's organization, by the way, helps anyone with disabilities.

Another milestone for me was that I started driving. My left bicep was still weak, and I needed a device to help. I steered the car with my left arm, and my right arm controlled the gas and brakes. I wasn't the best driver. In fact, when we were driving around Bethesda one day, I was taking a turn, and my left arm locked because of that little device. I ran over the median. But they were able to adjust my arm, and eventually I got better at driving. It's impossible to explain how losing so many things you loved and did before affects you, but with every little milestone, I felt more like the old me. Still, the "new" me, I realized, would be different.

But I had to keep moving ahead and making progress in all aspects of my life. Since I was getting pretty good at driving, we decided we needed a new vehicle, one that would accommodate a wheelchair. Someone suggested a minivan. Nope. Nope. Nope. There would be no way I could go from a two-door sports car to a minivan. We found a company that could do a truck conversion on a Chevy Silverado. Awesome. The VA gave me a one-time vehicle buying grant but that only covered $15,000. Semper Fi Fund covered the rest of the $40,000 cost.

I was back in the game!

My new truck was a beauty. My wheelchair fit right in the driver's seat. The driver's door and rear door were fused. All I had to do to open the door was hold a button to lower it, and when the door reached a certain point, it lowered the platform, allowing me to move my wheelchair right in. Then, a bolt under the wheelchair locked it into position so it wouldn't move as the ramp went up and down. And it was a trip trying to let Nasar decide what he should do. The first time I showed him the truck and the ramp, he looked at me as if he were saying, "What do you want me to do? Do you think I'm stupid or something?"

But Nasar was smart, and he caught on in only two tries. He figured out that when I opened the truck door and the ramp came down, it was time for him to get into the truck. I want you to know all this detail, so you can see that nothing is easy for quadruple amputees. Everything needs some adaptation and takes a while to learn and master. It is not for the faint of heart.

But the one thing that didn't get modified—unfortunately—was our formations. Every Monday, Wednesday, and Friday, we had to put on our shorts and t-shirts, stop what we were doing, and line up outside like sardines. Over sixty Marines were there. It was a waste of time. And if you are a staff sergeant or higher, you didn't have to go. There were times I didn't go to them. Not because I thought I was better, but it was just too difficult to get ready. After a bit, I was approached by a new Gunny, who I think was from Haiti and didn't speak the best English. He said, "Why aren't you at formation, Peck?"

"Why? Well, because there are times when I only get two to three hours of sleep," I replied. "Why don't you take ambien then?" he said, clearly annoyed. This guy really doesn't get it!

"Gunny, I'm not guaranteed eight hours sleep with ambien, and that could hinder my therapy," I tried to explain to him.

"Peck, you need to show up, and you need to start shaving," he continued.

I couldn't help it. I had to educate this dude. "Can I ask you how long it takes you in the morning to shave? I bet you're up and out the door in a half an hour max. Let me tell you, for me to get ready it takes at least an hour. It's not like I just wake up in the morning and leave. My mom has to get me up or I have to wake her up. I'm missing both my arms and legs, and I'm not sleeping."

I couldn't believe his response. "Why don't you just get a nerve blocker," he said. The dude had no medical experience, and all he wanted me to do is just to show up in formation. Stupid, stupid, stupid!

I was promoted to sergeant in May of 2012, which you would normally think is a milestone in your military career. What most people don't realize is that when you are a wounded warrior and promoted, it's not like they expect you to go to the next level as a Marine. It is a promotion in name only. But being an active duty Marine is not your job anymore. Your job is to go to your therapy and recover. Period. Plus, I was recovering at a Navy base, so what could they teach me about being a Marine anyway? And if you can believe it, my command was still busting my balls over idiotic things like shaving my stubble.

Anyway, I couldn't believe they wouldn't get over the facial hair issue! I get it. But it's not like I had a year-long beard. I think some of the Marines who have never seen combat don't always get what we're going through. But I made it my mission to not take any shit and support my buddies who were in the same position.

My buddy Adam Keys was great at that stuff, too. He was always trying to let the public know who we are and why we do what we do. Adam, a retired Army sergeant, is fearless. He's missing both legs and one arm and has endured some 200 surgeries. He almost died several times. But by the time you read this, he will have been to the summit of Mount Kilimanjaro.

One day, Adam's mom, Julie, invited me to this guy Scott Mallory's house. He has a nonprofit called Truckin' for Troops, where he drives guys like us to where we need to go. He hosts lots of outdoor events, too. He decided it would be fun to take us tubing on a lake. (Tubing this way involves a giant tube that gets pulled by a boat.) We put on our life vests and headed out on the lake.

At first, it was me and Adam and Scott's two sons. But at some point, one of Scott's sons wanted to get off. The boat came to a stop, and he got off. Sammy, Scott's daughter, hopped in and took his place. But when the boat took off again, I guess we all did not lean back hard enough. The front of the tube went under and the tube flipped, throwing us all in the water. Sammy, her brother, and Adam popped up. I didn't. Eventually, I did come up, but not before swallowing a fair amount of water. No more tubing for me.

As the months went on—remember, I was at Bethesda from August 2011 to November 2012—I had a Mother's Day gift to plan. Mom's old Pontiac was breaking down, and she was in the process of divorcing Gene. I wanted to do something special for her. "Mom, why don't I help you out with a new car, but you need to keep it below a certain price," I said. She cried. Soon she found a Nissan Titan, and I bought it for her. But I told her that was it for a while in terms of gifts.

Still, I realized my mom sacrificed so much for me. I soon scrapped that no-gifts thing and gave her two things she wanted on her bucket list. The first was a cruise to the Bahamas, which we took, and another was a trip to swim with the dolphins.

To do the dolphin experience, we went on a boat, then a small skiff until we got to the spot where all the dolphins were. On the skiff were a very nice couple and their six-year-old son. I noticed the boy was staring at me. No surprise there. It happened all the time. Finally, the boy got up the courage and said very politely, "Excuse me sir, what happened to your arms and legs?" Don't ask me why, but this is what I said to that sweet innocent boy. "Well, son, I was swimming in the ocean and all of a sudden a bunch of dolphins bit off my arms and legs." He looked at me in horror. When it was his time to be put in the water to touch the dolphins, he let out a blood-curdling scream. Oh my God, how could I have done that to this kid? I had no clue, but I felt really bad.

This experience, as well as my misadventures at the old Walter Reed, the Malone House, and now Bethesda, have taught me so many life lessons. At times, when people used to bitch and complain about their lives, I would think, *Yo, you think you have problems? Yours are nothing compared to mine.*

But the truth is that everyone has their own issues and handles challenges differently. My new attitude was that I would try to listen and be patient, and not give up on anyone who is lonely, poor, abandoned, or injured. It's the least I could do.

FIFTEEN

MAKING TRACKS WITH TRACKCHAIRS

BEING CONFINED TO A WHEELCHAIR IS NO FUN. JUST ASK ANYONE WHO SITS in one all day. For me, before my arm transplant especially, it was a complete pain. Sure, I had some fun racing my buddies in their wheelchairs in the courtyard of the old Walter Reed, but believe me, it's not what I had envisioned for myself. I was a cut, six-foot U.S. Marine, and tough. But now, with no arms or legs, I was afraid I would be stuck in this chair for life.

Like other things you get in the military, most are basic. The same goes for wheelchairs. That wasn't acceptable to me.

After I was feeling a little better, I decided that this wheelchair had to go. I had had enough. And so did some of my buddies. I was physically miserable sitting in that thing. I had to lift my stump up in an uncomfortable position, just to maneuver it. It became obvious that taking the wheelchair anywhere, except on a military medical base, just wasn't working. I realized that at some point, I had to talk about the situation with my command.

One day, Captain Woody was visiting Walter Reed and stopped by my apartment in Building 62 to see how I was doing. His real name is John A. Woodall, and he was the captain of a firefighter unit from Raleigh, North Carolina. After September 11, Woody and his guys traveled to New York City to assist his fallen firefighter brothers. He helped raise more than $7 million to assist the families of the fallen and even donated four fifteen-passenger vans that picked up their relatives, so memorial services could be held at "Ground Zero." Woody explained to me why the vans were so important.

He said that when first responders found a body in a pile of rubble, they sometimes couldn't bring it out because the conditions were just too dangerous. Since they could identify the bodies of firefighters by the name on their jackets, Woody believed that all his brothers should have a proper and dignified burial. Having vans available to transport the family to the site, he told me, was the least he could do to show his respect for their ultimate sacrifice.

Woody was also the driving force and project director behind raising money and building the North Carolina Fallen Firefighter Memorial in Raleigh, the capital of the state. He also started "Camp for Heroes," a great facility near Fayetteville, North Carolina, where guys like me and their families could spend quiet time relaxing, fishing, and taking in nature.

I don't remember the very first time I met Woody, but he reminded me of our testy encounter recently. Apparently, I gave him shit. I had just come out of my medical sedation and was feeling sick when Woody and some of his firefighter volunteers visited me in my hospital room. They decided to visit us wounded warriors at Walter Reed on a regular basis after 9/11 and after we went to war in Iraq. One time, I asked him why he wanted to get involved. He told me, "You guys are heroes and sacrificed your lives for our country. I wanted to do something to recognize that and show you all some love."

Woody got it. "John, the first time I met you, you had just come out of your sedation. I went into your room, and you kind of cussed me out," Woody told me. He could see that I was pissed and angry; I mean, who wouldn't be? I had just woken up only to find out that my arms and legs were gone. But Woody was cool. Since his dad was a Baptist minister, he knew just what to say. Plus, when he was an active firefighter, he was in a terrible explosion and suffered physically and mentally just like me. That's why I think he understood my feelings more than most people. All he said to me before he left my room was, "John, we'll pray for you; God is with you." That's how I first got to know Captain Woody.

Sometime around the summer of 2012, a guy named Kyle Johnson from Action Trackchairs, a Minnesota manufacturer, came to visit Walter

Reed. He demonstrated a Trackchair to us in the lobby of Building 62. I was totally intrigued.

Woody knew about my problems with the standard wheelchair. During one of Woody's frequent visits, I invited him over to my room and showed him the Action Trackchairs site on my computer. We saw that the company, in addition to making custom Trackchairs, also made specialized lifts for people who played golf. That's not what I needed. I said to Woody, "Hey, man, do I look like the golfer type?" He cracked up.

At the time, I was already in possession of some two-plus acres of land near Fredericksburg, Virginia, courtesy of Tunnel to Towers, who would later team up with Gary Sinise's foundation to build my smart home. A chair that could roll in the woods would be awesome.

We contacted Kyle Johnson, who was very open to the idea of customizing a chair for me. But there was a major problem. Each Action Trackchair sold for around $15,000. And insurance wouldn't pay for it.

Woody and I decided to contact Steve Danyluck, a.k.a. "Luker," the founder of the Independence Fund, a Charlotte, North Carolina, non-profit dedicated to improving the lives of wounded warriors. We showed Luker the Trackchairs, and he said, "John, count me in." The Independence Fund would help us raise the money and become a big part of the Trackchair story.

Woody and Jennifer also mentioned the chairs to Gary Sinise, and together they came up with a great plan. Gary's Lt. Dan Band was going to be performing a concert in South Carolina for the troops, and Woody asked the artist Scott Lobato if he would come to the concert and do a painting and auction it off to raise money for the chairs. (Scott was the guy who after 9/11 painted American flags in about five minutes.) Fortunately, he agreed.

Woody introduced Scott at Gary's concert and told the crowd enthusiastically and with the flair of an auctioneer, "You can take the painting home with you tonight and will be witnessing a national treasure unfold right before your eyes." By the way, Scott finished the painting while *God Bless America* was playing for the crowd. It sold for $20,000. I couldn't believe it! We were almost there. The next thing we knew, the guy who lost the bidding was so impressed with the painting and our mission that he told Woody and Jennifer that he would pay $15,000 if Scott would make him another painting just like the one he lost in the bid. That was a no-brainer. Thanks to this guy's generosity, we now had enough money to pay for not one, but two Action Trackchairs!

After the concert, Action Tracks began to work on our customized chairs and told us they would have them ready in time for Christmas. I thought, *That would be a way cooler Christmas present than the blanket I got as a kid.'* I was pumped.

Just so you know, for the past sixteen years, Woody and his nonprofit organization of firefighters organize and execute the biggest and best Walter Reed Christmas and Super Bowl parties ever. It's one thing we really look forward to each year. Woody is a great guy and helps people for all the right reasons. I say this because some so-called charities spend more on their salaries, fancy offices, and advertising than they do on helping the people they claim to serve. That's why we respect Woody so much.

To make the parties fun, Woody enlists his volunteer firefighters, and they come with all the food and gifts for the kids. Walter Reed provides the space in the Warrior Café, where the guys in Building 62 have their meals. The actor Jon Voight is a regular, and he always comes with gifts. Jennifer Griffin from FOX and her two daughters attend, as well as hundreds of the Walter Reed gang including us, the doctors, nurses, therapists, and many of our families and friends. There are also other nonprofits that always support Woody, including an amazing woman—Marie Bogdanoff—and her awesome charity called "Villagers for Veterans." Marie lives in The Villages, an adult retirement community in Florida. She decided to start a charity at the Villages to support wounded warriors and veterans by raising money for whatever they need. She even held one for me. (Did I mention that she is also disabled, suffering from polio when she was a child?) Marie is a saint.

At the parties, there is always entertainment. It's hard to imagine, but Woody does a damn good Elvis impersonation, even though he looks nothing like Elvis. Woody puts on his Elvis costume—with the wig and big sunglasses—and sings some of the King's greatest hits. It's ridiculous, but cool. I wouldn't do it, buy hey, you can't fault a firefighter for dressing up like Elvis and singing to a bunch of amputees. Right?

Sometime during the Christmas party, I'm not sure exactly when, Jennifer, Woody, and Luker surprised Adam and me with the very first Action Trackchairs customized for severely wounded warriors. I was embarrassed at first, but it was truly a great moment, even though we really didn't know how to work the chairs at that point. Adam and I almost crashed into each other at the ceremony. We had a lot to learn about what our new chairs could and couldn't do. They were very powerful machines. (In fact, after it was delivered to my home in Virginia, a buddy of mine came over, and we gave it a test run. We attached the Trackchair to his Ford Explorer, put it in neutral, and the chair pulled the truck up a small hill. Sweet! That's how powerful this thing was.)

But after Adam and I received our Trackchairs, it got me to thinking that all the guys who needed a chair should be able to have one, not just me and Adam. But at $15,000 a pop for the basic model, or even more for more additional bells and whistles, the cost could rise to $17,000. And who the hell would pay for them?

Over the next year or so, we literally created a Trackchair craze. Everyone wanted one. They were hotter than Hot Wheels. Jennifer talked to the former Fox News host and author, Bill O'Reilly, and he said he would donate $15,000 on the spot and would have the funds go to Steve Danyluck and the Independence Fund. Bill and Jennifer agreed that the Independence Fund would be a great charity to help raise money and present the official Action Trackchairs to the wounded warriors at Walter Reed and across the country. Luker was really pumped. He took the lead in helping organize our effort and was with us all the way. Did I mention that Luker was a former U.S. Marine and a pilot for American Airlines? Marines always are there for one another. Brothers for life. Plus, whatever any of us needed, Luker was the rock. In fact, after I decided that I could benefit from an "Endless Pool," where flowing water allows you to swim without needing a huge in-ground pool, Luker quickly agreed to pay for it. I said to him, "Luker, this is awkward." I was always uncomfortable taking things from people, but, in this case, I was happy to accept his offer.

Not too long after, Jennifer and Woody convinced Bill to come to Walter Reed. That way, he could see for himself what our Action Trackchairs were all about. About a week later, Bill, Jennifer, and Woody came to Walter Reed. Woody told me that Bill asked him, "What's the big deal about these wheelchairs?" Woody told him, "Bill, with these Trackchairs the guys could go anywhere they want. They can go to the woods and jump logs, drive through creeks and on frozen lakes or shallow streams, or climb up steep embankments. They can even go hunting and fishing and not get caught up in any rough terrain."

So, Bill O'Reilly not only had donated $15,000 for one chair, but promoted it on his television show and anywhere else he could. His national audience was so huge and loyal that in no time, the money was rolling in. (I think since he made that first visit to Walter Reed, he came to know our situation personally and stepped up to the plate even more to help.)

The Independence Fund, as well as Semper Fi, continued to promote our cause and raised enough money for any wounded warrior who wanted a Trackchair. Bill was so into our effort that he continued to promote our Trackchairs on Fox as well as his social media. He also decided to donate all the money from the sales of his best-selling books to the Independence Fund, the Fisher House, and others that help military members and their families. (The Fisher House, by the way, now has five facilities in the Department of Defense System. Like the Malone House, it helps families of wounded warriors being treated at Walter Reed by giving them a place to stay, and some of the comforts of home. The founder, Ken Fisher, established a foundation to keep the Fisher Houses afloat, and they have been a welcome respite for so many families like mine.) Despite his recent problems, I am still grateful for his contributions and passion for helping us gain our mobility. We couldn't have raised the amount of money we did without Bill.

It was another huge day when Bill decided to come back to Walter Reed to personally present a triple amputee, Adam Smith, with his very own customized Trackchair. Luker was there, along with Woody, Jennifer, Jennifer's two daughters, and many other supporters. It was awesome to see the look on his face when Adam got to sit in his very own, tricked-out-to-the-max, Trackchair.

Sometimes I can't believe how far we've come since that concert in South Carolina in 2012. With Bill's dedication, fame, and advocacy, plus Jennifer, Woody, Luker, and Gary's support, today the Independence Fund has raised a whopping $40 million for Trackchairs for wounded warriors. That means that guys like me—1,400 to be exact—now have customized Trackchairs designed to improve the quality of their lives. Though most of us still have serious physical and emotional challenges, and will for the rest of our lives, at least, thanks to the Trackchairs, our freedom is rolling along. I am so happy to know I played a part in the Trackchair project. It gave me even more determination to help guys like me get what they need to live the best lives possible.

Looking back, there were many things I learned from my time at Walter Reed, but among the most important was helping my fellow soldiers and Marines, whether with Trackchairs or, sometimes, just a visit to cheer them up.

SIXTEEN

NAVIGATING MY NEW SMART HOME

TRACKCHAIRS ARE GREAT, NO QUESTION. BUT EVEN COOLER WAS MY NEW smart home. For those of you who are not familiar with the term, smart homes are designed to help amputees and other people with severe disabilities to function on their own. Everything in the home is controlled by the brains of the operation, an iPad or a similar tablet. For guys like me, who after our injury relied on prosthetic arms or sometimes even arm stumps, all we do is touch an icon on the iPad, and it performs the task we want it to; that's huge. And I mean everything—lights, TV, security system. The warrior's dream!

But like a lot of big events in my life, I can't completely remember how the idea of my smart home got started. I learned later that Frank Siller and John Ponte, the guys I mentioned earlier from Tunnel to Towers, came with their wives to visit me in my hospital room at the old Walter Reed when I was still an inpatient. Tunnel to Towers is a foundation established to honor Stephen Siller, a brave New York City firefighter who died at the Twin Towers on 9/11.

They offered to build me a new smart home. I remember saying, "Yeah, that's great." But frankly, I'm not sure what I said. You have to remember I was totally drugged up in those days. But whatever I said, Frank and John had taken it as a "yes."

Betty was still with me back then, and we had started thinking about where we were going to live, if I ever got out of the hospital, that is. We knew we'd need help, so we started the application process for Homes for Our Troops, another nonprofit that builds custom homes for wounded warriors. One day, Frank and John came by again and noticed the application forms on my bedside table. "Hey, John," they said, "You agreed that we were the ones who were going to build your home, isn't that true? When we came by the first time, you were kind of out of it, but when we offered to build you a home, you agreed," one of them said. To be honest, I have no memory of that conversation.

But after my medical sedation was a thing of the past, I started looking around at smart home possibilities with a clear head. I decided it was a pretty damn good idea to go with Tunnel to Towers. At the time, they were building smart homes in conjunction with the Gary Sinise Foundation. Tunnel to Towers did the actual architectural plans and construction, and Gary's foundation raised money to build them through his fundraising concerts and private donations.

As Tunnel to Towers was beginning to plan my smart home, and even though I was still pretty drugged up, I started thinking about where I wanted to live. Naturally, my first thought was somewhere around Antioch. I looked up the number for the Illinois Veterans Administration and gave them a call. I asked about their prosthetics program. At the time, I was using a Bebionic arm, a British prosthetic that looks like the one Arnold Schwarzenegger left behind at the end of the first *Terminator* movie. I asked the VA if they could fix my arm if it broke. Well, it turned out they had no idea about Bebionic arms; they were still using lace-up prosthetics. So, Illinois was out.

Back then, my mom was dating a real estate guy, and she told him I was looking for land for my home. I decided I wanted to be near Bethesda, and I also knew they had a good VA hospital in Richmond, Virginia. So, it made sense to move somewhere in between.

This real estate guy helped us find a place. It was the first place he took us to, and it was in Fredericksburg, Virginia. We did our due diligence and continued to shop around, but most of the land we saw had houses right on top of one another. I really wanted a space where the neighbors couldn't see me, where I could ride around naked in my wheelchair if I wanted and no one would be the wiser. (Luckily for my new neighbors, that never happened.)

So, we went back to the Fredericksburg location, which is called the Estates of Chancellorsville, named after the famous Civil War battle that took place there. In fact, it turned out that the lot I was looking at had three

Civil War trenches right on the property. Nice to be a part of history, huh? I remember going into the model home to talk to the salesperson—they had to find a ramp for me, since the garage had only stairs leading into the home. I asked the woman how much a home would cost there. "About $1.5 million," she said. I almost shit a brick.

The $1.5 million, however, was for the model home, which had all the bells and whistles. My home would cost far less. The Tunnel to Towers guys took a look and agreed to the deal. By this time, their partnership with the Gary Sinise Foundation was in full swing. As Gary mentioned in his foreword, Hector Castro, the father of a fallen warrior, suggested raising funds for my home as a way to honor his son. A tribute to Hector's son was held in California and raised about $75,000. Eventually, through the efforts of Tunnel to Towers, Gary's Lt. Dan Band concerts—I went to one in Chicago—and donations from Operation Support Our Troops and Clint Eastwood, even more money came in. I was touched that so many people wanted to support me, and though I'm not one for a lot of personal atten-tion, I knew it was for a higher purpose. Plus, you have to remember that for guys like me with so many physical and emotional challenges, knowing we will have a permanent home takes one giant load off our minds.

We had a perfect day for the groundbreaking ceremony in early July of 2012, not a cloud in the sky. My mom was there with me, and so was Nasar. The folks at Tunnel to Towers and the Gary Sinise Foundation set up a little stage, and there were several reporters in attendance. I also remember there was a guy who was a Civil War reenactor. He showed up in full uni-form—Union, not Reb—and sweated like hell. Remember, this is July in Virginia.

A month later came the framing walk-through. John Ponte was there to meet me and my mom. So was Kristin Pruitt, whose family is the developer of the Estates. It was great! They had a big cardboard check for the home, and I gave it to Nasar to carry around. John asked me a lot of questions. He wanted to know where I wanted to put the TVs, for example, so that they could put in supports. In the master bedroom, I told them a wall needed to be moved to make the room bigger. Stuff like that.

My smart home was built fairly early in the partnership between Tunnel to Towers and Gary's Foundation, so they were sort of learning as they went. My fellow quad, Todd Nicely, already had his home built, but it would be several years before guys like my buddy Adam Keys got his. A lot of stuff was being done for the first time. For example, John Ponte had an idea for my shower that involved a wooden bench and several water jets. We found some Amish folks who built the bench from teakwood. I had three water jets for my body and a waterfall showerhead in the ceiling. There was also a flexible showerhead that I could use from my wheelchair.

I also talked to them about adding what I called a "pot filler" over my cooktop. Why this? Well, without a pot filler—which is simply a faucet near the stove that allows me to fill pots with water—I would have to take the wheelchair across the kitchen, fill a pot with water, and lug it back to the stove. They had already done the drywall by the time I thought of this, but Kristin Pruitt said it was a good idea. She actually wanted one for her house, too. So, they got it done!

They also put door motors over all the exterior doors. To open the doors, I had to press these handicapped blue buttons. I wanted to hide the buttons, but there was no way to do it. I also needed a fence around the house for Nasar. Kristin at first said that might be a problem. Visible fencing was not really allowed in the development. But we settled on a black chain link fence that was not visible from the street, so Nasar had his room to roam.

There were glitches, to be sure. All new construction has them. For example, the cabinets on the stove could be lowered with my smartpad, but they came down on top of the electrical outlets. I couldn't unplug the appliances before lowering the cabinets; my prosthetics simply couldn't do that. But like I said, this was in the early days of building smart homes. You just can't think of everything beforehand. But, no matter what, having a smart home, let alone one built by Tunnel to Towers and the Gary Sinise Foundation, was awesome. You can't imagine, unless you are missing all four of your limbs like me, just how hard life can be living in a house or apartment not designed for someone with my disabilities. The idea of a smart home for severely wounded warriors meant that now we can have a place built with our specific needs in mind. For example, everything, like I mentioned before, is controlled by an iPad or some other tablet.

With just one tap on my Samsung tablet, I could open doors and windows, turn on and off the lights, lower the kitchen cabinets, and so much more. I could turn on lights in parts of the house. I could control the TVs in the master bedroom, the living room, and the office. (My mom had a TV in her room, but I couldn't control that.) I could activate and turn off the security system and adjust the climate system. Out in back was a gas-powered generator in case the power went off. I could even lift the toilet seat. I could take my wheelchair into the shower. I just roll it right in. I can reach the washer and dryer doors, prep the vegetables right in my wheelchair too, and live as normal a life as possible. Each and every inch of the smart home is carefully designed to meet as many of the needs us quads have as possible—and like I said, while there is no perfect design, they are always trying to make improvements. Most of all, living in a smart home made me feel like I was back in the game. I could be semi-independent and begin to do the things that I did before—albeit without arms and legs.

It was really great that they involved me in all of the planning for my smart home, as well. I actually had a lot of fun picking out all the flooring and the granite for the counter and sink tops while I was still at Bethesda. Bassett Furniture agreed to completely furnish the house, which was so generous of them. I estimated that would have been an in-kind contribution of more than $150,000. They were also nice enough to let me go through the house room by room and use their website to select all of my furniture. The Bassett folks even showed up for my key ceremony once the house was ready for us to move in officially.

Speaking of which, what a day!

It was Veterans Day 2012, and the lead up to it was frantic. For one thing, I was getting shit from my gunny sergeant. What else is new? He insisted that I have an exit interview with the Battalion Commander, and he asked me what I want to do for a living after I leave the Marines. "Sir," I said. "I want to be a chef." If you can believe it, he told me: "Sgt. Peck, I will not let you exit the Marine Corps without a viable career option, and it's not like your hands are going to grow back and you'll be able to fulfill your dreams of being a chef." I told him, quite confidently I might add, that I didn't have to worry about a career because I would be financially doing very well, thank you, as a quadruple amputee.

For another, my mom and I had all this stuff in our little apartment in Building 62. After all, we had been living there for about two years. And it seemed like every time someone would come through, they would leave their own things, like pots and pans. So, we had to figure out what we wanted to keep, and how to get the rest of the stuff over to the new house. Fortunately, Dawn van Strike from Semper Fi arranged for some volunteers to pack us up and move everything down to Fredericksburg. My mom and I loaded up my truck with food and some remaining stuff, and off we went to my new smart home. It was a great feeling, and it was huge to experience something so positive for a change.

Just outside my new development, we met up with the Patriot Guard. These are guys on motorcycles—some ex-military, some not—who honor wounded warriors by forming a procession to escort them wherever they need to go. In my case, I was in the middle of a motorcycle parade leading right up to my new house. Pretty cool. And even though we did all this planning, I still wasn't really sure what the house would look like. I mean, I knew it was a white house with a blue slate roof and a red door, but I had purposely stayed away for a while, so I'd be surprised. Boy, was I psyched!

When we first pulled up, all I could see was this big American flag and a stage set up in front of my house for the ceremony. Once I got out of my truck, I found myself whisked off to the stage. There, I was in front of a crowd of some fifty people, including John Ponte, the Gary Sinise Foundation folks, and my man Adam Keys. Gary always stays away from these ceremonies, because he wants the wounded warrior to be the center of attention. He likes to visit the home when he can spend time with the new owner in a more private setting.

I nervously sat with my mom next to me on the stage as John Hodge, also from Tunnel to Towers, and Hector Castro made heartfelt speeches. I had a hard time controlling my emotions. After all, only two years ago, I was lying in a hospital bed, unsure if I would live or die, and if I lived, what my life would be like. I went through hell and back. I had my wife abandon me. I could hardly take care of my basic needs. Now, here I was, after years of intense therapy, sitting on a stage with my own smart home behind me. It was an enormous step toward my independence.

It was beautiful. It was a one-story contemporary home, with a white exterior and slated roofs. And it was all mine. When it was my time to speak to the gathering, I knew what I wanted to say. "I'm really not a hero," I said, as I looked out at all the people who got me where I was that day. "The real heroes are the people who didn't come back and who I think about each and every day. But I know they would be happy to see the generosity of people like you. A simple thank-you can't go far enough for what you've given to me today."

I really meant that. Keep in mind, for guys like me who have lost limbs, day-to-day living is a bitch. Things that most people take for granted— opening a kitchen cabinet door, putting clothes in the dryer, cooking dinner, or even taking a shower—can be grueling. Not to mention the time it takes just getting ready for the day. Before my arm transplant, I needed help with the simplest of things. For a quadruple amputee, a smart home is nothing short of a miracle.

I'd like to tell you a beautiful girl carried me over the threshold to my new house, but it wasn't like that. Actually, my first real look inside the house was kind of jarring, because all these reporters with their lights and cameras and tape recorders were right in my face. And as you know, I'm not a guy who's real comfortable with publicity.

John Hodge, the Tunnel guy, told me this was to be expected because it was my first day in the house and everybody wanted to get their stories done. But I also noticed one of my favorite new neighbors, little three-year-old Peyton, and her mom, Lisa, had come over to welcome me into the house and the neighborhood. So, I told those reporters, "Time out!" They had to wait to do any interviews with me until I had a chance to talk to Peyton and her mom.

The rest of the day was a complete blur. The officials sat me in front of the fireplace in my wheelchair. The goal was to have me available for interviews and whatnot. I talked and answered questions for what seemed like the rest of the day. We were also supposed to have a housewarming party, but one of the water lines broke, setting the party back a few days. Just as well. I was beat. I think I was in bed by nine.

Looking back, I was extremely grateful. I mean, I was still missing my arms and legs, but here I was, twenty-seven years old with a beautiful new smart house of my own and two acres to do whatever I wanted. And no mortgage, to boot!

But it was bittersweet, too, because I didn't know what the future held. I was now one helluva lot more independent, but for what?

In just a few weeks, I would be medically discharged from the Marines. I had this beautiful home, but no wife to share it with. And it was me and my mom again. I was happy she was with me, don't get me wrong, but a young guy should be living on his own without the support of his parents. Or in my case, just my mom. But I wasn't your regular Joe. I needed help and would for many more years to come.

And as for my last few weeks as a U.S. Marine, they were bittersweet, as well. Although I will always in my heart be a Marine, the last few months of shit I took from the Gunny sergeant had sort of closed the door on the Marine chapter of my life. I had mentally checked out long before leaving Building 62. But as with all major changes in life, you can embrace them and move forward, or go back to your dark spot. I had no intention of going back there.

My goal for my new future was to keep getting better and becoming more independent. It was also important for me to continue my support of other wounded warriors as well as single mothers and their children. And, despite my problems with relationships, I was hopeful that I would find love again, although I would do it differently the next go-around.

So, when the crowd all left, I went through the entire house, noticing all the cool things they had designed for me. I was truly moved. But the best part was my new kitchen. I told my mom to relax. Dinner was on its way. Though it took a bit to get used to the appliances, I got the hang of it pretty quickly. My first meal: leek and potato soup.

And once we were all settled, I actually put my plan into operation to do those random acts of kindness I told you about earlier. My buddy Mahlon Johnson agreed to help me, and we devised a pretty good plan to be executed during the Christmas holidays in 2012 and 2013. At first, we went to our local Walmart and asked to speak with the store manager. "Hey, we want to give single mothers gifts for their kids, and we want to pay for them." He seemed interested. "And it's not like we want to pay for expensive things, but for something a single mom's kid wants but she can't afford," I explained. I went on. "Sir, we have a couple of rules. The gifts have to be toys, no Xboxes and nothing ridiculously expensive." The manager pulled up three layaways, and we paid for all of them. I wish I could have stayed when they picked up the layaways to see the sheer joy on their faces.

Another time, I think it was Christmas, 2012, Mahlon and I went rogue and decided to go to Walmart kind of undercover and see if we could identify a single mother who looked like she might need some financial help. We spotted a woman who fit the bill, and I walked over to her and said, "Hey, my name is John, and I was wondering what you might need for Christmas. She was shocked. "Well, I don't have any good pots or pans," she replied. "Well, consider it done!" I found an awesome set of Paula Dean pots and pans, paid for them, and gave them to her. Just then, her husband came over, and she explained to him what we had done. While it turned out she wasn't a single mother, we still did a good deed, and that felt great.

I did many other random acts of kindness during those years, and it is so true about how it affects you. It takes you out of your own dark spot and makes you realize that almost everyone has some kind of challenge in their life. I may have no arms or legs, but that single mom might have been abused by her husband. The woman I gave the pots to may have had a terrible disease. Who knows? But doing things to help other people teaches you so many valuable lessons. Sometimes they stick and other times they leave you, but no matter what, it feels good.

And with all this going on, I didn't have that much free time, especially for meeting women. And with my track record, it was just as well. But, as I am with all things, I was not about to give up on finding a loving relationship. I'm a survivor, and even though I had two failed marriages, as they say, three's the charm!

SEVENTEEN

ALL ROADS LEAD TO BOSTON

S O, THERE I WAS, THE PROUD, MORTGAGE-FREE HOMEOWNER LIVING ON historic ground. Yeah, you might think that I would be psyched, but I still had no arms or legs. What would I do with my time? Fortunately, the answer came soon in the form of the Wounded Warrior Program, a state-funded organization in Virginia. (No connection to Wounded Warrior Project, by the way.) The program did things like organizing group therapy sessions for veterans, taking veterans to events, or sometimes just talking.

The coordinator for the program was a fellow named Mahlon Johnson. We didn't hit it off right away. In fact, I called him my "creepy little stalker" at first, because I soon found out he was driving by my house a lot and asking Kristin Pruitt about how I was doing. I briefly considered calling the cops. But one day, he stopped by and introduced himself. Lo and behold, he turned out to be a former Navy corpsman. Now you should know this: Marines love Navy corpsmen because they take care of us when we're hurt. (The Marine Corps has no corpsmen, like I told you earlier.)

Mahlon told me that he led a group that met every other Thursday at a local church. This was clearly a group therapy session. "If you wanted to come," he said, "just let me know." Well, I've never really been into that kind of thing, so I brushed it off. I tossed his card on a table near the front door and forgot about it.

Mahlon would figure prominently in my life, but I didn't know it at the time. I had bigger fish to fry, namely, getting my new home in order. One of the first things I did was head to Bed Bath & Beyond and drop $3,000. I bought pots and pans, kitchen appliances, knives, forks, spoons, baking sheets, a mixer, a blender, a Keurig coffeemaker—you name it. My mom and I spread it all out on the kitchen floor—it filled the whole room—and I took pictures. The aspiring chef was in business, even though my right arm was useless, and my left was just a hook.

Then it was on to the backyard. As you'll recall, it was fenced in for Nasar, but there was no grass. When it rained, the yard turned to mud that Nasar never failed to track. I tried seed, but it didn't take. I decided to pave over about half of it and use it for an entertainment center, complete with a stone fire pit and seating area.

As I was planning all this, Dawn Van Strike, from Semper Fi, happened to call. "How's it going?" she asked. I told her about the backyard, and before I knew it, Dawn said Semper Fi would foot the bill. "John, let us help you; we're happy to do that," she said. I don't like asking people for help, and, besides, Semper Fi had already helped me with buying my first truck after I was blown up. But Dawn can be persuasive. Long story short, I sent them an invoice for a nice stone patio. And it was paid in full.

I also happened to notice Mahlon's card one day. I looked it over again and figured what the hell, why not call? I did, and Mahlon told me they had a fishing trip to Beaufort, South Carolina, coming up. I passed on that one, but Mahlon called me later about another trip to a private lake in Virginia. "John, do you want to come?" he asked. "Hell, yeah," I said, "But, dude, I can't handle a fishing rod." He said, "John, don't worry, you'll have a fishing buddy to do whatever you can't." So, I ended up going, and Mahlon ended up as that buddy. I used that Greifer in my right hand to hold the rod, and to my surprise, I ended up catching a nice large-mouth bass. In fact, I caught more fish that day than anyone else on the trip. Go figure.

As it happened, Mahlon and I were becoming friends. And Maj. Jim Hoover, who you'll remember as the guy who got me the Tom Brady game jersey signed by all my beloved Patriots, moved to Fredericksburg with his wife and two daughters. He and I became friends, as well. Slowly, my Virginia circle of friends was expanding. It felt good.

Mahlon even persuaded me to attend his group therapy sessions. He said it wasn't because he thought I was suicidal or anything, just that he thought I might be able to help some other warriors who had issues. "Some just can't get past the PTSD," Mahlon said. "John, I think you could be a big help to them. Some guys just can't get over it, and others don't even try. And there is another Marine who is always complaining, and I think he could relate to you." So, I agreed to go. Mahlon said he would pick me up and take me over.

I never spoke during my first visit; I was just there to help.

I still remember this one guy who came in limping, with a cane. He was all upset because, he said, one of his guys got hurt in the field. "I wish I was with him," he said, "I don't know if he'll ever recover." Well, it turned out that this guy was in the Marine Corps Band, and the "field" he was referring to was the marching field. He even complained about a sore back from carrying a tuba. You can imagine what I—a fucking quad injured in combat—had to say to this guy.

But other guys were more serious, and so were their injuries. There was this one fellow with PTSD who didn't want to go to the VA because he thought it would somehow take funds away from guys like me. I told him that's not true. The fewer the guys who go to the VA, I explained, the more the VA's budget will shrink over the years. He finally went and got help. He even got a big chunk of back pay. I gotta say, I felt pretty damn good about that.

Still, I have to admit I was getting bored during this period. Yeah, I had Mahlon and Jim Hoover as buddies, but I didn't know anyone else. My house was about twenty minutes from downtown Fredericksburg, just long enough to be a hassle. So, to occupy myself, I came up with the idea of a saltwater aquarium. I bought all the stuff—a fifty-five-gallon tank, lights, sand, rocks, a filtration system, the works. I also bought some fish from a local store and actually ended up volunteering there—talking to customers, doing this or that—two or three days a week.

I also got to be the honorary captain for a basketball game at a local private school, courtesy of the younger of my buddy Jim Hoover's two daughters. The game came with a bonus: one of the team captains was a fellow named Brent Hunsinger, who owned a local landscaping company. It felt good to be out in public, making new friends in the neighborhood and trying to get back to a normal life. To me, these seemingly meaningless and everyday experiences were monumental. They gave me a slice of my old life back, and I was going to take all of it in.

Brent and I would become buddies, too. He ended up doing the landscaping for my front yard and designed a tropics-like enclosure around my pool in the side yard. (I swam in that pool every day for months leading up to the operation. I had to strengthen my shoulders.) I came to trust Brent; he would later look after my house while I was in Boston. But doing something major about my condition was never very far from my mind; I guess I refused to really believe that I would be a quad for life. I had previously met with a doctor at Johns Hopkins in Baltimore, but he felt that my left arm, because of the fungus that ate my bicep, would not be a candidate for a transplant. So, I kind of buried the thought for the time being.

But the truth was that I couldn't let it go. It kept eating at me, and I knew I had to keep searching to find a solution to getting my life back. In November of 2013, I decided to do a computer search on a guy in Spain who received a double leg transplant. This time, the first thing that came up was Brigham and Women's Hospital in Boston. They were looking for candidates for a double leg transplant. Naturally, I started going through their programs; the more I saw, the more I liked. I quickly scrolled down to the bottom of their page to find a contact. I was psyched.

The contact person was a woman named Lisa Quinn. I promptly wrote her a long email, explaining that I saw they were looking for a double leg transplant candidate and I might be interested. I asked for more information so I could decide whether to toss my hat into the ring. Hey, I even emailed her photos of my amputations. Trust me, they weren't glamour shots!

I didn't hear back for a while, so I literally called her at least three times a week. My persistence paid off. Finally, I heard back from Lisa in early December. She said the doctors would love to get me up to Boston, but it was getting close to Christmas and New Year's. So, she suggested we wait until the new year; we scheduled my visit, which included a week of testing, from January 7 to January 15.

I headed up to Boston the day before my testing was to begin. The trip was eye-opening in a lot of ways. Right off the bat, it introduced me to what would become a major issue for me—money. Most people are under the misguided impression that we wounded warriors are loaded. Rich, that is. The truth is that no money in the world could compensate us for what we lost. From limbs, vision, and independence—to husbands and wives, and what it does to your mind and soul—believe, me, it is no picnic. Not only all of that, but once you are disabled, you are rated on what type of injury you have. That determines your annual disability payment. And if you are an amputee like me, you are given a lump sum on top of that disability. So, for example, a missing arm can give you a lump sum payment of $50,000, two arms, $100,000 and so on. While that total compensation package might sound like a great deal, it comes with a steep price.

Traveling to Boston, however, upped the ante. The hotel tab for that week—nothing fancy, no Ritz-Carlton for me—came to a whopping $4,000. Another $2,000 went to renting a handicapped accessible van. And that's not counting the food. Ouch. But I was determined to see it through.

Lisa was waiting when we arrived. She took us up to a small conference room on the hospital's second floor, and there they were—a group of doctors and surgeons who, although I didn't know it at the time, would change my life forever.

I was greeted by Dr. Bohdan Pomahac, the director of plastic surgery at Brigham and Women's Hospital. He introduced me to Dr. Simon Talbot, an unassuming New Zealander who is director of the hospital's upper extremity transplant program. Then all the doctors began to parade past me. There was an immunologist, a kidney specialist, an infectious disease guy—fifteen doctors in all! Before I knew it, they were all talking to me, laying hands on me, testing my range of motion. "John, we need to run some tests on you, but how do we draw your blood?" one of the doctor's asked.

That was a problem. At Walter Reed, I had a PICC line. (For you non-medical folks, that's a peripherally inserted central catheter, or a line into my blood system that can be used for a prolonged period of time.) But I hated the one at Walter Reed, because the nurses scraped my bone with the needle when they put it in. Trust me, that's not a feeling you ever want to experience.

At Brigham, they first tried to get blood through the scars on my left elbow. No dice. In fact, I yelled at a nurse when she probed my elbow for a vein. But they had to figure out a way. The doctors were worried that the flesh-eating fungus might still be in my tissues, on the theory that my immune system had figured out a way to keep it dormant. They also were concerned that I had developed weird antibodies from all the shots and blood transfusions I got in the military. If that was the case, I could only accept limbs from a donor with the same antibodies. Good luck with that.

Finally, they decided on a subcutaneous power port, which is a tiny plastic gizmo embedded just below the skin in my chest. It's connected to the main artery leading to the heart, so to get blood, all they need to do is put the needle into the port. But it took some getting used to. I'm a stomach sleeper, and it's a challenge to sleep that way with a piece of plastic in your chest.

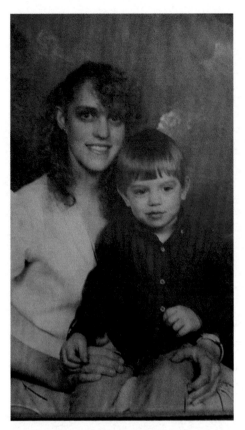

Norma holding John in a formal portrait as a young boy. *Peck family photos*

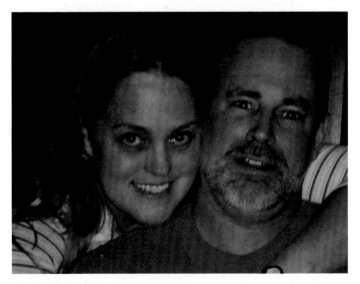

Uncle Toby and Mom. *Peck family photo*

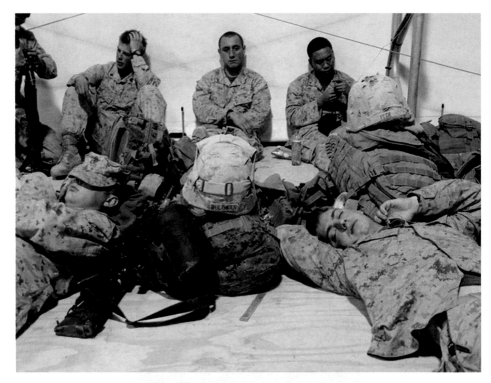

John in Afghanistan. *John Peck*

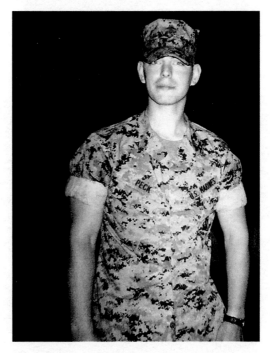

Lance Corporal Peck reporting for duty. *Peck
friend's photo*

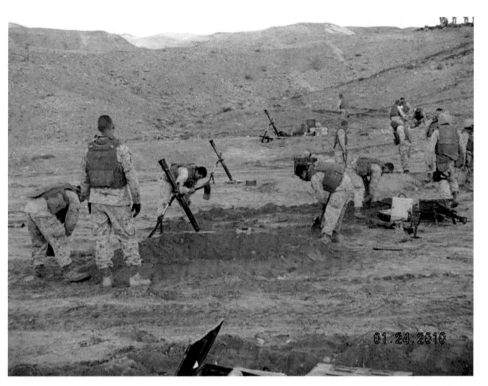

Mortar gun line. *John Peck*

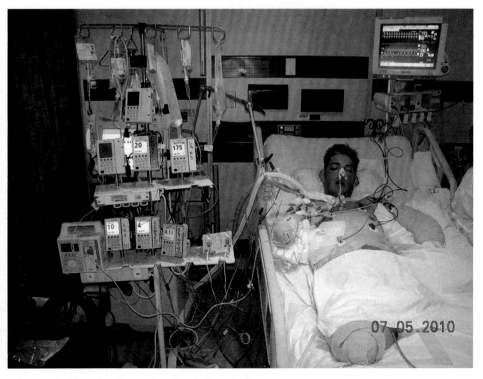

John medically sedated at Walter Reed. *Peck family photo*

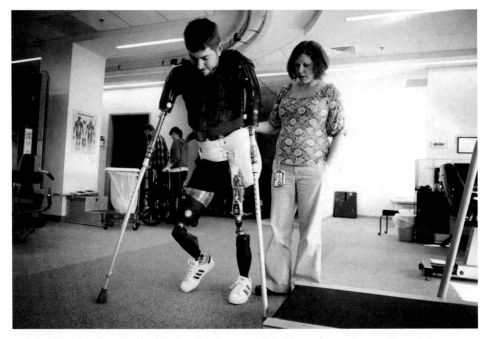

VA physical therapist helps John to walk. *Hillary Swift from the* Freelance Star

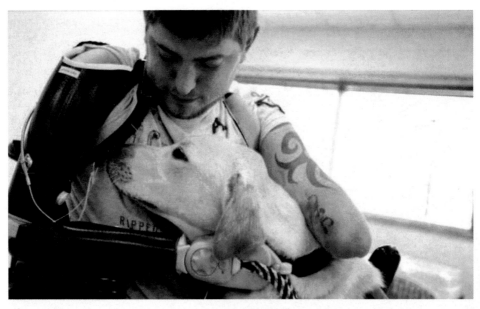

John and Nasar meeting for the first time. *Peck family photo*

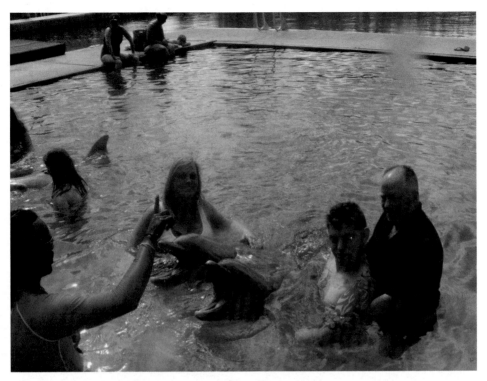

Norma and John swimming with dolphins. *Peck family photo*

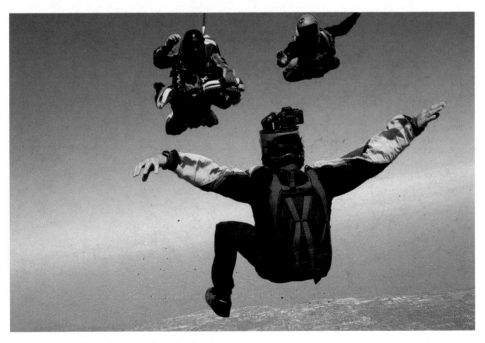

John does his first sky dive. *Peck family photo*

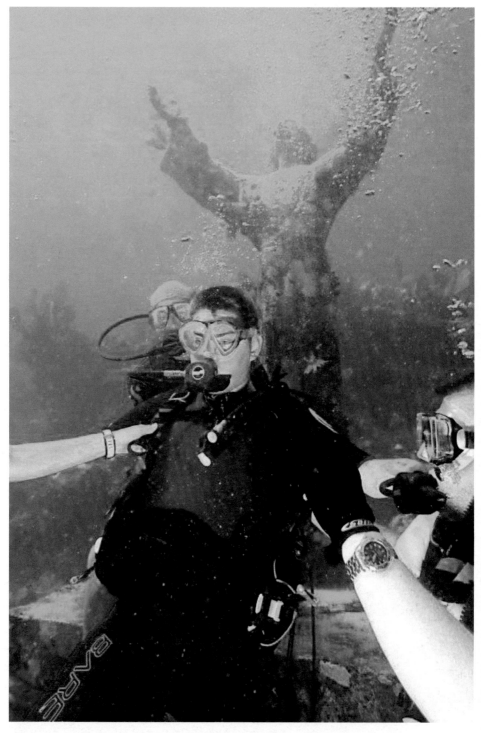

Who says a quadruple amputee can't scuba dive? *Peck family photo*

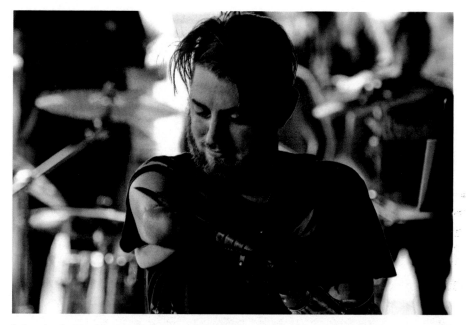

John checks out his new body-powered arm that can be adjusted manually to control its grip strength. *Rebecca Cunningham Photography*

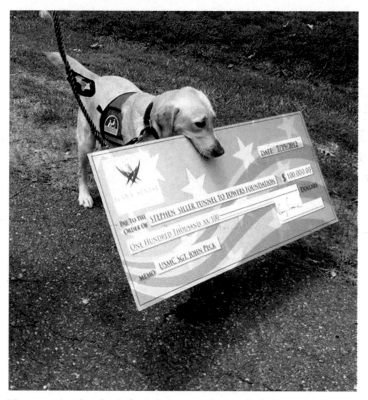

Nasar carries the check for John's smart home. *Peck family photo*

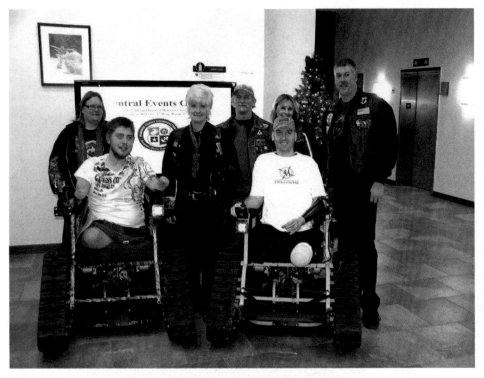

John and Adam Keys (right) receive the first Trackchairs. *Peck family photo*

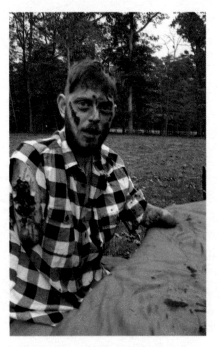

John dressing up as a zombie on Halloween. *Peck family photo*

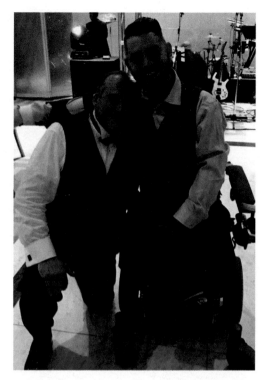

John and John Ponte from Tunnels to Towers at John Ponte's daughter's wedding. *Peck family photo*

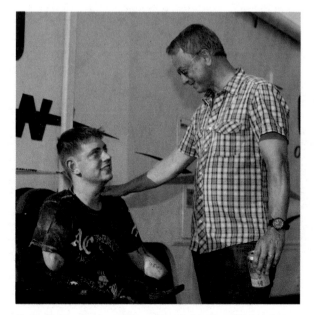

Gary Sinise, actor and founder of the Gary Sinise Foundation, visits John in the hospital. *Peck family photo*

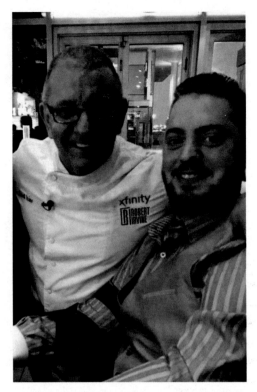

John and his friend and mentor, Chef Robert Irvine. *Peck family photo*

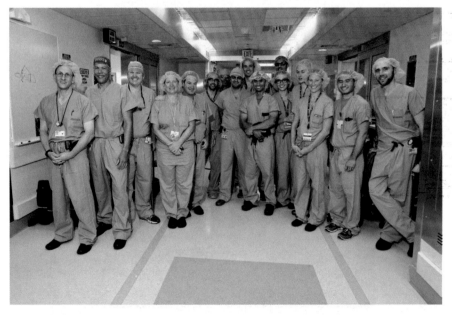

The amazing surgical and medical team at Brigham and Women's Hospital. *Brigham and Women's Hospital*

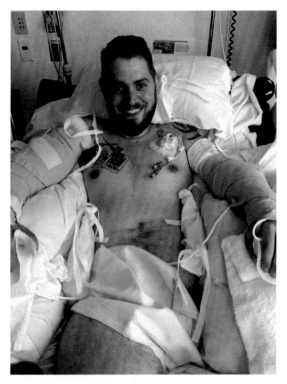

John right after his bilateral arm transplant at
Brigham and Women's Hospital. *Jessica Peck*

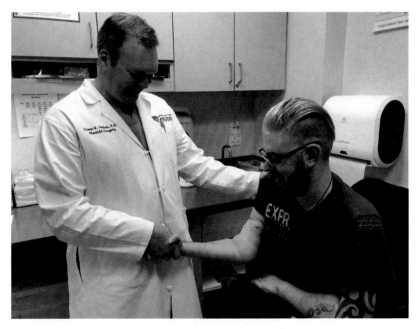

Dr. Talbot and John shake hands for the first time. *Jessica Peck*

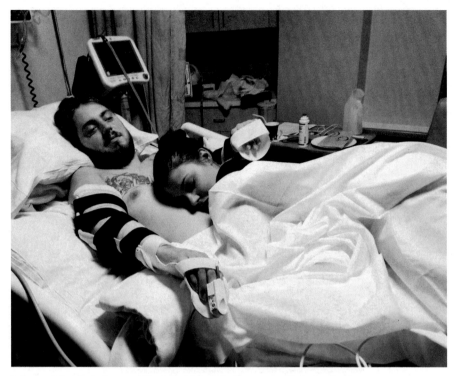

John and Jessica's first cuddle following John's surgery. *Peck family photo*

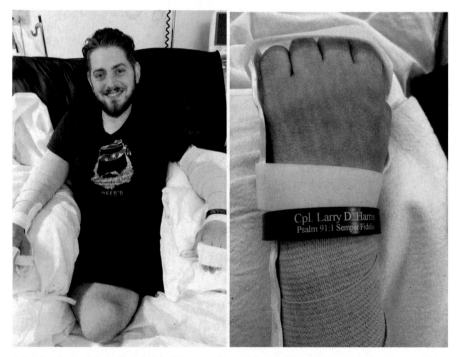

John finally is able to honor his fallen buddy, Cpl. Larry Harris, on his new donor arm. *Jessica Peck*

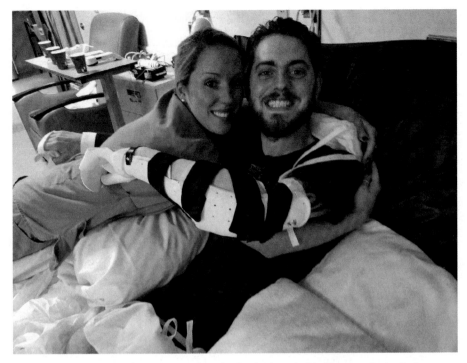

Nurse Katie and John share a hug at last day in the hospital in Boston. *Jessica Peck*

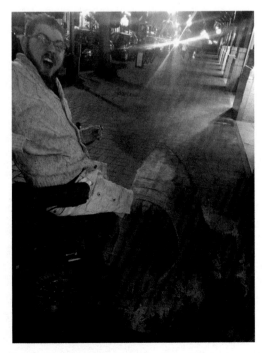

John showcasing his amputee humor in
Victoria, Canada. *Jessica Peck*

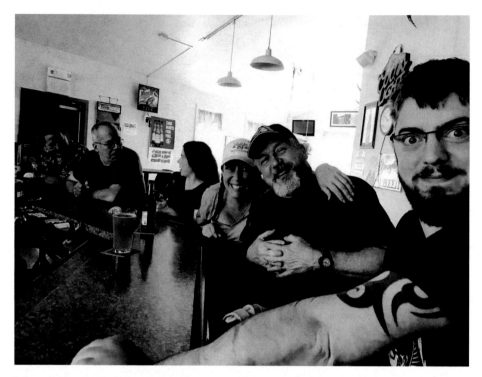

John meeting Jessica's family for the first time. *Peck family photo*

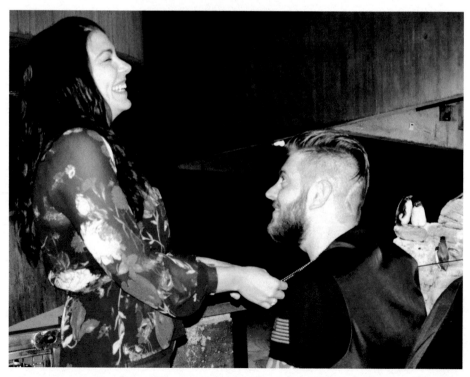

John proposes to his girlfriend, Jessica. *Abi DeLuca*

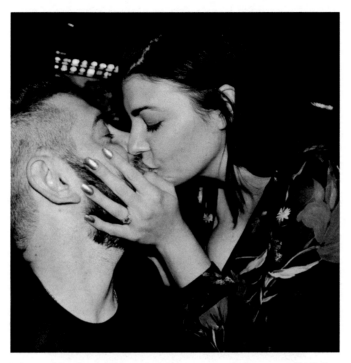

John and Jessica celebrate their engagement in Boston. *Abi DeLuca*

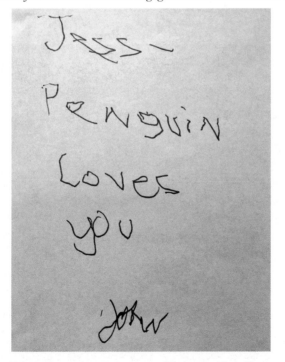

John's first written message to Jessica for their first wedding anniversary after receiving his donor arms. *Jessica Peck*

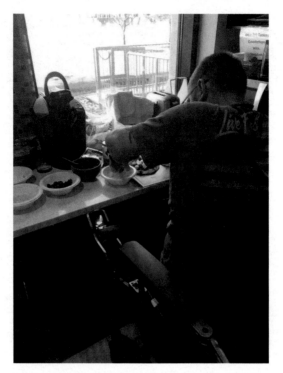

John cooking pizza following his arm transplant. *Jessica Peck*

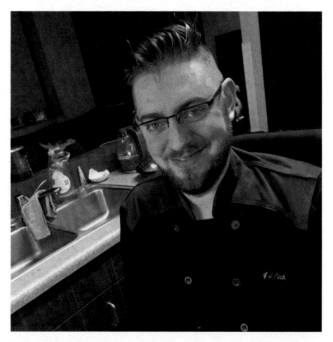

John in his chef's jacket, ready to prepare Jessica's Valentine's Day dinner at Walter Reed. *Jessica Peck*

Meanwhile, the tests continued in different parts of the hospital with Lisa Quinn at my side for everything. One test I remember was when they used a catheter to do an angiogram. For that one, I wasn't totally under, just sort of semiconscious. I remember the machine above me as they went in through my femoral artery in my leg and injected dyes. Basically, they were making sure my body could handle new limbs and that my heart could supply enough blood. They also got a road map of which arteries and veins were present to join to my new limbs. They did a psychological test, too, to make sure I understood and could handle everything that would happen to me after I receive someone else's limbs.

I had no idea at the time how emotional that would be.

At the end of the week of testing, I sat down with the doctors. "You know, John, we need to sit down as a group and decide if you're a good candidate. We'll base our decision based on the testing and your personality. A lot more goes into this than you think," one of the doctors told me.

One of them—I can't remember which one—had mentioned to me at the start of the week the possibility of an arm transplant. Because of that left leg disarticulation, they reminded me, a leg operation would be very difficult. I knew that already. But then Dr. Talbot stepped up in front of the group and asked in his distinctive Kiwi accent, "We want to do your arms, then we'll see about your legs. Are you okay with that?"

"Like, hell, yeah," I replied. "But remember, John," Dr. Talbot said, "This is still very preliminary. We need to look at everything and make the decision at our next team meeting."

It turned out the next meeting at Brigham wasn't until February. Waiting a month was agony, but I used the time to do more research on this Dr. Talbot. It turns out that he is a world-renowned transplant surgeon who has done four double arm transplants and two others like mine above the elbow. (I learned later that with his disarming—see what I did there?—manner and expressive green eyes, he's a big favorite at Brigham. It turns out he once tried to reattach a woman's nose after a pit bull bit it off. He persuaded a local police chief to pump the dog's stomach, find the nose, and rush it to the hospital. Sadly, it didn't take.)

The call came on February ninth. "John, you're accepted as a candidate for surgery. Congratulations," they told me. I am in! The feeling I had was a combination of excitement and relief. I was thrilled that my dream of receiving a donor's arms was going to finally become a reality and, at the same time, relieved that the anticipation was over. I took a long, deep breath. It was the beginning of a journey that would take me to a place I could never have imagined.

But there were some conditions. They needed some unusual things. Like, they wanted me to see a dentist in Virginia to make sure there were no weird diseases in my mouth. They also needed a form certifying that my blood was B Positive. They needed a better psych exam. Oh, and they told me I had to stop smoking. They would later test to make sure I was free of nicotine.

I called Keith Borders, one of my case managers from the Hunter Holmes McGuire VA Medical Center. He wanted me to drive to Richmond for the dentist appointment, but I didn't want to drive an hour and a half when I could see a dentist right here in Fredericksburg. (Thankfully, because of the Veterans Choice Program, that's now possible.) The verdict: I had no weird diseases, only the gingivitis I picked up in Iraq. But I still had to make the drive to Richmond for the psych exam.

I would say the psych exam, more precisely a neuropsychiatric test, was more like an intelligence test. Its purpose was to see if there were any problems resulting from my TBI, any changes in the way I thought or felt. I guess they wanted to make sure I understood what it would be like emotionally—waking up with someone else's arms attached. I nailed the answers right away. The guy who did the testing said, "Well, you're not crazy. In fact, you have above average intelligence. The only thing we found was that you're slow to admit your faults." "Not true at all," I said.

Once all the testing was done, my mom and I decided she should have her own place. She had given up everything to take care of me after I was blown up the second time and deserved some time on her own. Luckily, my mom found something about twenty minutes away. I'll admit we had a few spats about when and how long she would come over. After all, my mom was still being paid by the VA as my caregiver—which is how the VA compensates all military caregivers—but there were still a lot of things I couldn't do by myself. But we worked it out. Like, on days she couldn't come over, she would set up things for me, like putting the mug on the Keurig and placing my meals in the microwave.

The silver lining, though, was the fact that her absence forced me to become much better in doing things for myself. For example, when I dropped my phone, Nasar would always pick it up. But, of course, he would sometimes scratch the screen, and he always slobbered on it. So, I learned how to lower my wheelchair, gently slide to the floor, and pick up my phone. Then I'd grab a pillow, prop myself up, and crawl back into the chair.

Animal lover that I am, I also got a German Shepherd puppy. I called her "Athena," after the Greek goddess of wisdom. I soon learned how to open the kennel for her and how to get on the ground to scoop food into hers and Nasar's automatic feeders. I even figured out how to plug in my phone to recharge. Thanks to all these factors, I felt that I was becoming increasingly more independent. Finally!

Meanwhile, I still had a ton of questions for the doctors in Boston. The main one was, would there be a place for me to stay during and after the surgery? They told me they didn't have one, since I would be their first out-of-state patient; there was no long-term housing available. They were nice enough to contact my insurance company to see if they would pay for the operation, but they said no, too, because the surgery was considered experimental. Fortunately, Brigham and Women's Hospital decided to absorb the cost. But the hotel was still on me.

I also had to worry about how to get there. I decided to take a hard, realistic look at that major issue I mentioned—money. I sat down by myself, looked at all my bills, my monthly income from the VA, and all the new costs I'd incur from the operation. These were big. I'd need to stay in Boston for three to six months following the operation, then return to Boston every quarter for the first year. After that, visits would be twice a year for five or six years. That's one hell of a lot of hotel, van, and travel expenses, including paying for my mom. Not to mention food. There were other costs, too, like putting Nasar and Athena up in a kennel while I was away.

After an epic math session, I came up with a good estimate of the total cost for my part of the operation: $400,000!

Of course, I didn't have that kind of money. But I did know a guy, Alex Marrocco, the father of Brendan Marrocco, the first quadruple amputee from the Iraq War and the first military guy to get a double arm transplant.

Alex told me I needed to set up a trust fund. He contacted a local lawyer and filled them in. They were great, did it all pro bono, in fact. But I had to make some hard decisions. There had to be a trustee. This would be the only person with access to the account. I chose the one person I knew I could trust, my buddy Mahlon. There also had to be a death beneficiary, even more important than usual for someone like me facing major surgery. I picked John Ponte, from Tunnel to Towers.

Then came the hard part. Raising money. First, I began laying out my problem on Facebook and created my *John Peck's Journey* Facebook page.

It generated a little social media momentum. Then I set up a website, JohnPecksFund.org. I had t-shirts made up, so people could buy them on the website or just donate. I set up a PayPal account, too. Everyone who either sent a check or a made a PayPal donation got a thank-you email from me. Every single one.

Before too long, I started getting some media attention, not all of it positive. For example, some people accused me of fraud. They assumed the VA would pay for everything and that I was simply trying to get money for myself. Seriously? I had to explain that the VA wasn't paying for anything, other than my monthly check. Let's just say I got a good education in the downside of social media.

My big break, though, came on Memorial Day of 2014. I still don't know how it happened, but I was selected to appear as an honoree at the traditional Memorial Day concert on the National Mall in Washington, hosted by actors Joe Mantegna and Gary Sinise. That would mean national attention for my cause. I asked them if they could include my website on the broadcast, but they said they couldn't. But they did put it on their website, which was awesome.

From that day on, I was off and running. When I got back to my hotel that night, I had over 200 emails, almost all of them notifications of donations! The vast majority came from regular folks across the country and not large organizations. That made me feel great, knowing that my fellow Americans cared enough about a total stranger to donate their hard-earned money to me. Thanks to the concert and the media attention that followed, I eventually raised $450,000.

What a relief! With the money taken care of, it was time for me to consider the logistics. The doctors at Brigham told me that timing was everything. From the time they identified a matching donor, I would have only eight hours to travel from Virginia to Boston. Otherwise, no good. The eight-hour deadline was now in my head 24/7.

I knew a guy who worked for Operation Airlift Command, an organization that puts wounded warriors in touch with people who own their own jets. I told him what the situation was, and he put me in touch with the CEO of Jet Blue Airlines. Jet Blue was great. They gave me multiple company contacts—no way I wanted to get voicemail when I called—and guaranteed me a seat on any of their flights to Boston. I stayed in contact with them through this whole thing. (In fact, the Airlift Command guy also set me up with a Vietnam veteran in Dallas who founded a company that loans money to veterans. Talk about doing a fellow veteran a solid: this guy had his private jet pick me up at an airport near Fredericksburg, take me to a buddy's wedding in Texarkana, and fly me home. And he would have flown me to Boston had the call come in while I was at the wedding.)

The only thing dicey about the travel arrangements was Brigham's insistence that no one—well, only those who absolutely *had* to know—be told of the reason I was flying. There were good reasons for this. For one, let's say I told someone who knew someone in the media. Then maybe there would be a media mob at Brigham. For another, the doctors wanted to make sure I survived the operation and there was no rejection of the new limbs before declaring a success. Finally, remember that for me to receive new arms, somebody had to die. Out of respect for the privacy of the donor and his family, they wanted the date of the surgery to be kept private. So basically, just Mahlon, my mom, the folks at Jet Blue, and Brigham knew.

So, everything was all set. But I still had plenty to worry about while I waited. What if the call came at midnight, and there was no scheduled flight available? What if it came in the middle of a snowstorm in Boston? If that happened, I'd be out of luck.

And, of course, even if the transportation went okay, what if the donor's arms didn't take? What if I didn't survive? These questions haunted me day and night. But strangely, at the same time, I was filled with excitement. The prospect of petting my dogs. Cooking my dinner. Maybe even taking a shower all by myself. It was all going to be worth it.

EIGHTEEN

FINDING MY PENGUIN

WHILE ALL OF THIS WAS GOING ON, SOMETHING JUST AS COOL WAS happening. I was in the process of falling in love with a woman who would become my wife.

Here's how it happened: In the early part of 2016, I was thinking about getting off Match.com. Unlike some folks, my profile was totally honest. I told people I was a Marine who was injured in Iraq and Afghanistan and lost my arms and legs. But, truthfully, that got me nowhere. Most of the women I was interested in had no interest in me. I would write to them, and they would delete my email. Not great for my self-esteem.

Then one day, something wonderful happened. A woman named Jessica had seen my profile on Match. She was interested. In fact, she sent me a Facebook message. She said she had just moved to the D.C. area. She said she had studied anthropology at the University of South Florida in Tampa and was well traveled. *Hmm*, I wondered, *was I on to something?*

She said she thought my Match profile was funny; she said she loved my sense of humor. I mean hey, who wouldn't like to get to know a quadruple amputee with a wicked wit? I think I had a few impressive lines like "I'm a blast to be around." (By the way, some of us amputees enjoy sick humor about our disabilities. Some of the things we say would totally freak a lot of people.)

It turned out Jessica had checked me out thoroughly before that first Facebook message. She checked to make sure my profile photo from Match was the same as the one from Facebook. She saw that I had friends on Facebook, and she went through my posts. Only then did she finally message me on Facebook.

Her message was sweet, but at first it sent up a red flag for me. Some of the messages I got were scams, and I was tired of dealing with them. Like, some chicks were what I called "camera models." You click on their link, and they get naked for you. My first response to Jessica was "Hey Creeper."

I left Jess's message alone for a couple of hours. By midday, I went back to her message, and I noticed she had looked at mine. *Maybe she's not one of those random chicks*, I thought. That was a good sign. I responded with a heartfelt message explaining that I'd been burned before. She was so sweet; she understood.

At some point during our marathon messaging back and forth, I said: "Hey, I don't mean for you to think I'm trying to do a booty call or anything like that. But I would love for you to come over, and we can sit around and talk if you like." She agreed; I immediately gave her my address.

My potentially *normal* date was on her way! As she pulled off Interstate 95 on the way to Fredericksburg, I called her and said, "Hey, is there any way you can pick me up a Monster drink?" Jess was more than happy to oblige. She stopped at a local convenience store and then drove into my development. It was very dark, and there were no street lights. Driving at night, it felt like you were in the deep woods, like a scene in a horror movie.

The house was so new that there was no GPS to guide Jess to the exact location, so we did it by phone. (Oddly enough, that was the first and last time she ever got cell phone service in my neighborhood. Must be fate!) I turned on every outdoor light, so that Jess could find her way. I waited outside for her, even though it was so cold I could see my breath. Finally, she pulled up in my driveway and emerged, wearing a maroon sweater dress and black UGG high heel boots. Surprisingly, our first meeting wasn't awkward at all; I gave her a huge hug.

When we got in the house, she opened the Monster drink for me and grabbed a straw. We stayed in the kitchen talking for about an hour. "John, can we sit down?" she asked. "Oh my, sure we can," I said. We walked—or at least she walked—over to my large blue couch, sat down, and we continued talking. We had a few drinks. She was so sweet and really interesting. It occurred to me at that moment that this woman just might be the real deal. After we finished the last drink, I moved closer to her and put my left arm around her shoulder; we kissed.

It was a great moment. In fact, over the next few months, as we got to know each other better, we had a lot of great moments. Like the first time she stayed over. Gentlemen and Marines never kiss and tell, but what happened the next morning was too good not to share.

At 10:00 a.m., the doorbell rang. We were still in bed. *Who the hell is that?* I wondered. I told Jess to stay in bed while I checked. It was the maids. (I love Nasar and Athena, but dogs can dirty up a place in a hurry.) After letting the dogs out, I let the maids in but told them not to go in the master bedroom.

Meanwhile, Jess was getting out of bed. She put on one of my shirts. Her dark, long hair was tasseled like an unraveled ball of string. (Sorry, Jess, that's the way it was.)

I decided to make us breakfast. I put some bacon in the pan on the stove. My mom had cracked some eggs for me the day before, so I went to the fridge and grabbed two more for Jess. Even cracked them myself and picked out the shells. Jess and I were talking when I smelled something weird. The bacon was burnt to smithereens. (A word about my bacon. As an aspiring chef, I take great pride in making my own. I would go to the butcher shop and get the best seven-pound cut of pork belly. Then I'd brine the meat for seven days, then add honey and brown sugar and put it in my electric smoker for another fourteen hours. Using her professional deli slicer, mom would slice up the bacon and divide it between me, her, and my buddies—Jim and Brent. My bacon is as close to culinary heaven as you will ever experience. But thirty seconds too long in the pan, even the best homemade bacon will burn.)

Despite the fact that we couldn't get our forks through the charred meat, we tried to eat the bacon with our eggs. But then the doorbell rang—again!

"What the hell is going on?" I said to Jess, as she looked at me in bewilderment. I got up from the table, opened the door, and there was my "DISC," the acronym for a Marine who helps me with anything related to the Marine Corps. He was a captain named Mark Beasley, and he was with a woman I didn't know. (Wounded warriors get several levels of protection to make sure their needs are met. There is a federal recovery coordinator whose job it is to tie the VA and DoD together. She was my bridge. I also had a case manager who just helped with the VA.)

"Hey man, did we have an appointment?" I asked Mark. "John, I'm here to visit and check in with you. This is Mrs. Lawrence, by the way, and she heard about you and wanted to meet you in person and see what you need," he said. Mark is great, but I wasn't really in the mood for company then.

I thought, *This girl stayed the night. Now the maids are here, I burned the frickin' bacon, and now these two people.* Then all of a sudden, I saw a big red Nissan Titan roll up the driveway. It was mom. "Hey, guess who else you're going to meet today," I said to Jess, attempting a feeble joke. But actually, I was seriously pissed! My mom wasn't supposed to be there. Since she was my caregiver, she didn't need to knock on the door; she would just come in. But why of all days was she here now?

So, there we were on our first morning together—the maids, the DISC, the other woman, mom; and then there's Jess. *This seriously isn't happening,* I thought.

"Mom, uh, this is my friend Jessica," I said, as she was eyeing Jess up and down, the way only mothers can do. I sensed the tension in the air. Mom sat down at the dining room table with Jess and me. The DISC and his friend, thankfully, left. Then my mom began her military-style interrogation.

"So, who are you, and how long have you been talking to John?" she asked Jess. My heart sank. I was afraid my mom would freak Jess out, but their discussion was surprisingly cordial. Disaster averted.

We had other misadventures, as well. After a few more times at my house, it occurred to me we should go out on a "proper" date. "Jess, I think we're skipping a step," I said to her one night on the phone." "I think we need to go on a date to a really nice restaurant. What kind of food do you like?" She told me that she loved Parisian food. Luckily, I found an awesome, accessible French restaurant right in Fredericksburg. I made our reservation for 6:00 p.m. Jess left her apartment in Arlington at around 4:00 p.m., thinking that would leave her plenty of time. She also had a bottle of wine with her. What she didn't realize was that traffic on I-95 South is horrible around that time. I know firsthand, since I had to drive that same route when I needed to have blood drawn every six weeks in preparation for my arm transplant.

At 5:30 p.m., she called me in a panic. No way she was going to make our first "real" date. Three hours later, she finally arrived at my house and said she was sorry. "I didn't want to show you how upset I was, but I was freaked out," Jess explained. We made it to the restaurant by 9:00 p.m. Jessica was driving, of course. But she forgot to bring her identification, so there were no drinks at dinner. The restaurant ended up comping us for the meal, but I had no cash for a tip. Jess covered it, but I felt bad because I wanted to pay for everything.

We had a very intense conversation that night. In my heart, I knew she would be the soul mate I'd been searching for all my life. I told her, "Jess, I've been burned so many times, I didn't think I could ever meet a woman I could trust again." What she said to me touched my heart. "I've been hurt too, John. But one of the things that impressed me about you was that even though you've been burned, you were still willing to give it another shot. You're willing to try love again." That really made sense to me. Here we were, two peas in a pod. We were two wounded love warriors, but we never wanted to give up hope. I'd like to think I put her heart together again that night.

Over the next few months, we had plenty of dates just like that. We laughed, we cried, we cooked. She told me that she loved the fact that I would make her a home-cooked meal. I asked her what food she missed the most. My luck she said, "John, I really miss beef tartare." *Oh, shit, this is going to be hard,* I thought.

"Don't worry, Jess, I got this," I told her, wondering how the heck I would be able to put that dish together. But after three days of research, I found a great recipe for Parisian beef tartare. I even bought stainless-steel ring molds. I planned to serve it with *pommes frites*—that's what the French call French fries—and a Caprese salad, a simple Italian mix of sliced fresh mozzarella, tomatoes, and fresh basil. I went to the local butcher shop with my mom and bought a filet mignon. As I've said before, it sucks to have someone drive you all over the place at my age—especially your mom—but it's all part of learning to cope on an everyday basis with a disability like mine. I'm happy to report that Jess was impressed with my culinary efforts. Not only did I create an authentic beef tartare for her, but I found beef she felt comfortable eating. After that night, I knew Jess was the one. Someday, I was certain, she would become my wife. About a month after our official first date, I went to the mall with my mom. I wheeled over to the Zales and started looking at rings. "You're not thinking about proposing to Jessica, are you, John?" she asked. I couldn't believe it. "Hey, I'm how old again, Mom? I'm an adult, and I can do what I want. Yep. That's it." I asked her to leave the store. She walked out and found a bench to sulk on. I know my mom was just trying to protect me. After all, she didn't know Jessica from Adam, and I got that. But I saw in Jess something I hadn't seen in a woman since Darlene. And that was her caring and nurturing personality, and an abundance of empathy.

I found the perfect ring, which I intended to let Jess know was not a marriage proposal but a "promise ring." Jess came over the next night. I had it all planned, as any Marine would. I ordered flowers and lit candles so when she walked in those would be the first things she would see. "How the hell did you light these candles with no arms, John?" she said. I gave her a long answer, complicated enough for a diagram. She made a face; we both cracked up. Nothing is ever simple for a quad.

We went into the dining room, and there on the table was a basket I made with her favorite flowers, some lavender items to help her with her insomnia, and some other stuff for her new apartment. Then she saw my promise ring in a small, nicely wrapped jewelry box. I asked her, will you be my girlfriend? Yes, she said.

She would also be my "penguin," and I hers. She had called me her penguin before, but I always thought it was because I waddled when I walked. "No, John, I called you *penguin* because when emperor penguins find their soul mate, they mate for life," Jessica said. *That was a relief*, I thought.

As the weeks and months went on, Jess, my penguin, got to know my friends and went with me to a few events as well, including a fundraiser organized by Jim Hoover and Brent to help people afford their private school tuition, as well as a wounded warrior motorcycle ride in Virginia, where I was the beneficiary and even got to give a short speech to an appreciative audience. I was happy that Jess fit right in.

One hot Thursday morning in August, Jess was in Arlington on her way to work. I called her as usual. She was rushing but told me, "Hey, John, I've got a work meeting, and I'll be back in about an hour. Love you; talk to you later." Later that day, I was sitting on my couch with Nasar and Athena watching TV when my phone rang. The number had a Boston area code, but it was a number that I didn't immediately recognize. The folks from Brigham would call me periodically to do a "checkup." They would ask me questions like "Do you still want to have the transplant, John, and if anything's changed, what's your plan?" I would tell them that nothing has changed.

But that day, I somehow knew the call was not just about a checkup. This was *the* call; I just knew it. I was downright giddy as I answered the phone. "Hello John, this is Dr. Talbot. Don't freak out, but I think we have a donor." I was speechless. "But don't do anything yet, John, just have your plan in place. Our initial testing looks good, but we have a few more things we have to do," he said. "I need to know now if you're on board." I looked at my watch. It was 4:00 p.m. "Yeah, Dr. Talbot, I'm still good. Let's do this," I told him.

I was already thinking of how I would get to Boston as we continued the conversation. After I hung up, I literally started bouncing around on the couch, as much as a guy without arms and legs can bounce. I was beyond excited.

Then it hit me. Worse than if a truck ran over my dogs. I lay down on the couch and started crying. I was happy, but at the same time, I knew that someone died. I was crying with joy and gratitude for the fact that the donor's family was willing to do this selfless act. Still, I felt terrible for this family even though I didn't know who they were or really anything about them.

After I composed myself, I picked my head up a bit, and the next thing you know, Nasar, who never cuddles, came up to me on the couch and put his head on my chest. Athena is the jealous type, so she couldn't resist joining the party. She came over too and laid her head gently on the other side of my body. They were so in tune with me, and it was comforting to have them around, especially that day.

About five minutes later, I thought, *That's enough; time to go.* Another Marine tactic. Switch gears and implement a plan. I immediately called Jess. She didn't answer. I sent her a text in all capital letters asking her to call me ASAP. She called me back a minute later. I told her we had a match. "You're kidding right?" Jess asked. "What does that all mean?" I told her we still had more testing that needed to be done on the potential donor, but it could be a few hours or thirty minutes. "You go back to work, Jess, and I'll let you know."

I called my mom, but she didn't answer. Finally, I got hold of her. "Okay, John, are you kidding or are you serious?" she asked me. I've played that trick on her before. "Is it time? I'll be there in a few minutes," she replied. Next, I called Mahlon. I told him I had a potential match, so I might have to start spending money. As my trustee, only Mahlon could transfer funds into my other account, the one I could use.

Then I called Andrew from Operation Airlift Command. "Dude, I don't need the flight just this second," I said, "but can you start looking?" The final calls went to Jim and Brent, who would be looking out for my house.

Mom finally arrived. We got together all the things I needed. Dr. Talbot called me back at around 7:00 p.m. and simply said: "John, it's a match!"

The words I was waiting and hoping to hear for so long!

Then I called Jess, who by that time was at her apartment, packing up. I told her to get an Uber and meet us at the airport. Mom drove me to the airport. It was an hour drive but felt like the longest drive of my life. We met Jess there; my mom cried and hugged me for a very long time. I was in Marine mode, stone-faced and intent on the mission ahead.

Previously, we'd agreed that for the operation I would go by myself. Once I knew I would become an outpatient, within two weeks my mom would come. She would put the dogs in the kennel, and Mahlon would make sure all the nonessential electrical stuff at my house would be shut off.

Jess insisted that she go with me. Fine. She didn't want me to be alone. I was so grateful I had such a strong support system. I had heard through the grapevine that another person waiting for a transplant couldn't get one because they didn't have that support system. That's crucial for success.

As we were sitting in the terminal, I kept thinking that my second wife abandoned me after my second injury, and a woman I only knew for about five months wouldn't leave my side. My girlfriend did more for me in that short time than my wife ever did in years of marriage.

I couldn't wait to hold Jess's hand.

NINETEEN

My Bilateral Arm Transplant: The Run-Up

THE STAGE WAS NOW SET FOR THE MOST IMPORTANT DAY OF MY LIFE. IT unfolded with all the precision of a well-planned Marine campaign. In fact, it was set in motion well before I received my fateful call.

Dr. Talbot had emphasized that there would be a whole team of experts involved. For example, Dr. Chandraker would manage the cross-matching, Dr. Blazar would attach the bones on my left arm, Dr. Caterson would join the blood vessels on my right arm, and so on. I had my own team of Brigham "All Stars"!

In the wee hours of that same day, while I slept with no thought of Boston on my mind, a call from the New England Organ Bank—now New England Organ Services—had come into Brigham and Women's Hospital. "We may have a suitable pair of donor arms here," the hospital was told. The arms were from a young man who had died of a brain aneurysm.

The wheels began turning. Within an hour, Dr. Talbot was awakened with the news. The doctor was told that the family was willing to donate their son's arms—nothing is possible without this consent. Testing began almost immediately at the hospital where the donor lay. So many conditions had to be met. Did the blood type match? Was there an immunological match? Did the skin colors match? Could the arms be removed at the same

time as the other organs? Were there any abnormalities? The list was long—
Dr. Talbot, I later learned, had a reputation for being very "choosey" when
it came to donor arms.

As morning broke, the meetings began at Brigham and Women's—the
surgeons met, as did the anesthesiologists and nurses. They had to make
sure an operating room was available. Luckily, all the key players made themselves available. They assigned a surgeon to each of the four arms—the
donor's pair and mine. It was a total team effort.

The donor's family officially gave the organ bank consent to remove
the arms in the early afternoon. Dr. Talbot and his team examined the lab
results from the hospital where the donor was—the hospital was relatively
close—and determined that the donor arms would be acceptable. Dr. Talbot
then placed that fateful call to me.

A couple of hours later, Dr. Talbot convened the entire team at Brigham.
The list was pretty darn impressive: orthopedic surgeons, plastic surgeons,
transplant surgeons, anesthesiologists, infectious disease specialists, radiolo-
gists, social workers, psychiatrists, nurses—to name just a few.

The team had planned and practiced these operations so often that the
meeting mainly served to confirm what they had already planned. They ran
through a PowerPoint presentation of my details, those of the donor, and a
timeline. Each team member got a checklist of what he or she was expected
to do. If it sounds by the book, it is—but only to a degree. Dr. Talbot said
these meetings always have an almost electric undercurrent of excitement
and anxiety.

As all this is happening at the hospital, Jess and I arrived in Boston
around midnight. After some snags at Logan Airport—the joystick on my
wheelchair got broken on the flight, Jessica ran out to meet the hospital
folks and couldn't get back through security at first—I was put on a gurney,
and we set out for Brigham.

Although we were in an ambulance, the entry to the hospital was strictly
stealth. We went in through the back entrance. Then it was up on the elevator to a pre-op room, me still on a gurney. Jess had rushed packing to the
point that some of her clothes were still wet. She hung them up to dry in
the bathroom.

Before long, the tests and questions began. They were pretty basic. Had
I been sick? If so, the operation might be off. I had not. Dr. Talbot came in
and inspected my arms, making sure everything was okay. They took some
blood and hooked me up to an IV; I was incredibly excited.

As all this was happening, I overheard someone saying that the Brigham team had left to pick up the donor arms. All I can say is that it was weird and at the same time exhilarating. But the fact remained that after all that I have been through—two blasts, loss of all of my limbs, and all the personal stuff—this moment would be the most intense of my life. Very few people in our country and around the world know what it is like to lose so much and potentially have so much to gain. In only fourteen hours, I would be joined with a stranger, and he would be the reason I would become almost whole again.

With all that racing in my mind, I don't know how, but I managed to fall asleep for just a few hours. Around 8:00 a.m., Dr. Talbot came in to see me, accompanied by a Brigham video crew. He checked me over and told me they were going to put nerve blocks in my shoulders. Those are injections of local anesthetic—the needle guided by ultrasound—to deaden the nerves in my arm stumps. It hurt like hell. But by this time, I was no stranger to pain.

A couple of hours later, the nurses arrived. "John, we're going to be taking you right in to the operating room," one of them said. I was scared shitless. I couldn't hug Jess because of the nerve blocks, but I told her, "I'm fine. I can do this."

Jessica hugged me as they wheeled me toward the operating room. I remember turning my head back to see her. As the nurses turned the corner with me, we both started sobbing. Jessica was crying, too, and my nurse, Lisa Quinn, gently approached Jess, gave her a gentle hug, and took her to the surgical waiting room. Later, she even called for a car to take Jess back to the hotel to get some much-needed sleep.

We both knew it could be our last time together if things went wrong. It was gut-wrenching.

In the operating room, they placed me very carefully on the operating table. Dr. Talbot touched my shoulder and told me to sit tight—that there would be a little wait time. Then, they began hooking me up to the heart monitors. Can you imagine my emotions during that gap between me being prepped for surgery and it actually beginning?

This is it! I thought as I was lying on that operating table. *Six years after I stepped on that goddamn IED and two years after I started down the transplant path and Jessica and I made the mad dash to Boston, here I am, on the table, waiting for the arms that belonged to someone else.* So many things raced through my mind. I could have arms again. I could cook. I could hug Jessica. I could be almost whole again.

Then in a split second, my mind turned dark. *What if it doesn't work? What if after all this, all the tests, all the travel, all my fantasies about having arms again, the surgery goes bad?*

I'll admit, I totally lost it. My head felt like it would explode, and I started sobbing yet again. What if I died on this table? This wonderful nurse, Jocelyn Lin, began to place the mask on me. She leaned down, touched her forehead to mine, and said, "Don't worry, John. We're not gonna let you die."

As I gazed into her eyes, ready to respond, I was out.

Several miles away, surgery began on the donor arms—one surgeon for each donor arm. The tendons, nerves, muscles, and blood vessels were freed and labeled. It was a painstaking, two-hour process, much of it done with loupes, which are powerful magnifying lenses on glasses. The arms were flushed with a solution of heparin and saline and filled with a preservation solution. Then they were placed in a large cooler filled with ice; the team left for Brigham with both of my donor's arms in tow. It was showtime!

TWENTY

THE TRANSPLANT ITSELF: REARMING A MARINE

S HORTLY AFTER NOON IT WAS SHOWTIME! I WAS OUT, OF COURSE, UNDER anesthesia. So, the following account is courtesy of Dr. Talbot.

The first order of business for the surgical team was basically a "time-out," to make sure everyone knew the plan to the most minute detail. Then I was prepped and draped to ensure sterility. Then the team began to reopen my arm stumps. By the way, each of my arms had an identical surgical team working on them in total unison. Dr. Talbot had warned me many times that this surgery would be very complicated and difficult. After all, it's not as if my arms had been neatly removed; they were ripped off by that stinking IED. But despite that, the surgeons got it done by fully opening each arm and basically recreating the wound.

Then, using their loupes and a big suitcase-sized microscope on rollers, they carefully began attaching these little waterproof tags to all my important stuff—my arteries, veins, nerves, muscles, and tendons. Each one was labeled, and the labels matched up with the tags that the other surgeons had meticulously attached to the donor arms. Dr. Talbot joked it was kind of like painting by numbers. "We don't want any confusion about what goes where," he said. This process took two surgeons about two hours on each of the four limbs. Before it ended, my surgery required a total of twelve surgeons over fourteen hours!

As they were completing the tagging, the donor arms arrived in the operating room. Packed in ice in a cooler, they were pale and cold to the touch, the little tags clearly visible. The operating room went silent, I was told, as the donor arms were brought in and put in position. Had I been conscious, I would have surely detected the excitement in the room. Hey, I would probably be jumping up and down. "It's really an exciting moment when they bring in these beautiful arms," said Dr. Talbot. "Super-exciting, really."

The bone work came first. As Dr. Talbot told me earlier, connecting my arm bones to the donor's provided stability for everything that came next—kind of like the scaffolding on a building. This was done very carefully. First, stainless steel plates were attached to my arm bones and those of the donor. Then they drilled tiny holes in the bones and inserted stainless steel screws. Everything had to line up just right—from matching the rotation of the bones to the length of the arms themselves. It's a painstaking process. This was only the second above-the-elbow transplant ever done by the Brigham team. Once the bones were together, out came the large microscope. Then began the exacting work of connecting all my blood vessels to those of the donor arms. There are large and small arteries, different types of veins, and their job is to supply oxygenated blood to and from the extremities. (I should have been a doctor.) They do all this by lining up the blood vessels in tiny clamps and then hand-stitching the vessels together with nylon sutures the width of a human hair. Can you believe that? On the other hand, the veins have floppier walls, and the surgeons used a tiny device called a "coupler" to join them—a plastic ring with spikes on it that hold the two ends together.

This part of the rejoining procedure required tremendous concentration over roughly four hours. Since the surgeons have practiced this over and over, they prepared for any eventuality as well as their own fatigue. They rotated in and out of the operating room as they got tired.

Dr. Talbot told me that at this point in my surgery, my donor's arms were still not functional. Each arm had all the blood vessels connected, but there were tiny clamps, so no blood was flowing yet. I'm no surgeon, but even I know that without the blood flowing, nothing works.

Now comes the magic moment. I was AWOL for this, of course, but here's how Dr. Talbot described it:

"The most exciting part is when we removed the clamps. Now the blood is flowing in and out of the arms. For about thirty seconds, we saw the waves of red spread down John's arms to his fingers. The donor arms, cold and white when they came in, were now pink and warm. We were literally watching John's arms come back to life," Dr. Talbot said.

"This is the magical part of the procedure," he added. "Many of us have spent months—even years—preparing for this moment, and now it's here. The entire operating room was silent. It was amazing!"

For the next hour, they added redundancy; more blood vessels were joined. Then the team joined the nerves. With nerves, they had to make sure the orientation was correct. "Special care must be taken with the nerves, which resemble wet linguini," Dr. Talbot told me later. "The bundles of neurons in the nerves must line up exactly, or else the new arms won't work."

After ten hours of intense concentration, the surgeons reached the final stages. Now the muscles and tendons were joined, and the big microscope was taken away. Surgeons then began to tailor the skin. They kept lots of extra skin to allow for swelling. They also attached external monitors for stuff like blood flow. The biggest fear post-op is that a clot will develop. When they monitor, they get a warning and can go back in and quickly correct any problem that might arise.

By midnight, it was almost over. The doctors trimmed off some excess skin. The surgery was now complete. I was officially rearmed.

I went into the operating room around 10:00 a.m. on a Friday; it was now 2:00 a.m. on Saturday. I should mention that a surgeon was texting Jess every two hours during this whole thing. And the Fisher House Boston was nice enough to take her to a Morton's The Steakhouse to eat and back to a hotel to get some sleep. But she couldn't. Jess would end up awake for literally forty-eight hours. I would say that would be tough even for a Marine like me.

Finally, I was wheeled into the intensive care unit, still connected to all kinds of tubes and monitoring machines. Dr. Talbot had called Jess just after the surgery and told her to come back around 10:00 a.m. Then he called her again a couple of hours later and said, "But don't do anything to stress him out." As if she could ever be the cause of stress.

I was groggy from all the medication but was able to respond to some basic questions. "John has taken on real purpose, a real sense of responsibility to the donor to make the most of this opportunity," Dr. Talbot told Jess. "This has taken away his disabled persona, and he never took on the role of victim. John determines his own future," Dr. Talbot added. I was moved by his words when I heard what Dr. Talbot said.

I really woke up around 10:15 a.m., gagging on the tube they were pulling out of my throat. Now they wanted to make sure the blood was flowing well, so they cranked up the temperature to well over one hundred degrees. I was sweating like crazy. They let Jess use a cold, wet cloth to help me cool down. What I wouldn't have given for a Gatorade at that point! In addition, I had this really painful pressure spot on the back of my head. That was because my head was propped up and immobile for about sixteen hours during and after the surgery. I remember the first thing I said to Jess when I actually could speak was "I told you I could do it. I got hands." I kept saying that over and over.

And speaking of the hands, my first thought was, *My God! Dr. Talbot has given me baby hands!* I guess it was the drugs. But Jess convinced me they were not baby hands at all; they looked fine.

And they were! After the baby hands scare subsided, I began to examine them with Marine precision. It wasn't weird psychologically; I accepted them from the start. But it was nevertheless a surreal experience. My only negative thought was that they had taken some of my left arm stump off to make things work. I worried that if my body rejected the new arms, I would be left with even less of my left arm.

Jess sent individual messages to Mahlon and my mom. She also sent a group message to Jim and Cheri Hoover and Brent and Beth Hunsinger when my anesthesia started wearing off and asked them if they wanted to talk to me. I remember speaking to Brent and Jim. They said everything was fine at home.

My mom decided to stay in Virginia. I obviously needed help, so after a long discussion, Jess said she would stay and help me after I was discharged from the hospital. Jess never helped me with any of my trips to the toilet before, so I knew it might be weird for her. And it was. But she rose to the challenge, and in a strange way, it made us even closer. Hey, if someone is willing to wipe your butt, they must be pretty cool.

The first night after surgery was bad. My body kept pushing the nerve blocks out, and the pain was incredible. Over the next two-and-a-half weeks, in fact, they had to reinsert them four times on one side, three on the other. That first night, the pain was so bad that I was literally minutes away from begging the team to reassemble and take my new arms away.

But then, I thought about the donor and what he had to sacrifice for me. I thought, *I will never give up on this young man who gave so much to me.* I hunkered down and somehow got through the night.

I worked through the misery, though it wasn't easy. Before I was me—Sgt. John Peck—and now I'm sharing part of my body with a stranger. I told Jess about this odd feeling, too. They tried to reassure me that I was still the same person I was before the surgery. But I wasn't. So much of my body was lost, but now parts were replaced, but they weren't mine. Who owned my new arms? Was he a good guy? As I looked down at my fingers, which were very stiff and not functional, I saw that he and I had a lot in common. We both had long, thin fingers, a similar skin color, and most of all, the right amount of hair. He and I were now one.

I got to thinking more about my donor. Here I was with his arms, and he was gone. It's like getting an unexpected chunk of money after a lawyer reads a deceased person's will. Only in my case, I wish I had known who my donor was and been able to say "thank you" to his family for his sacrifice.

By this time, I was completely aware that these are enormous operations and the likelihood of something going wrong was inevitable. There will always be complications, but you have to plan for them. It's like building a house. You can anticipate a lot, but you always have to be on the lookout for faulty wiring, problems with the framing, and all the other unforeseen possibilities.

But so far, so good. There were no immediate rejection symptoms. Dr. Talbot had told me that the first few months or so would be crucial to make sure that my body wouldn't reject my donor arms. The team would monitor me closely every day for about a month. Dr. Talbot and his team had to be prepared for anything.

"No one can do everything," Dr. Talbot said. "I am the director of upper extremity transplantation at BWH and have been involved with four transplants here and one at another hospital. None of these is easy. As we do more, we will get better. We learn something from every operation we do. I can tell you that John's case was one of the more difficult ones because of his wound. What was left after the blast was not a normal, clean-cut wound. But John is literally the most determined person I have ever met."

You got that right, doctor!

TWENTY-ONE

THE LONG, HARD ROAD
OUT OF BOSTON

THE DAY AFTER SURGERY WAS BETTER, THANK GOD. THEY INJECTED NERVE blocks, so the pain was minimal. I continued to worry about my left arm, but all in all, everything seemed smooth, and even their protocols were reassuring.

Before I would leave Boston, six tough months would follow. But in the days following the surgery, the therapy began almost immediately. There were lots of stretching exercises and lots of moving my (or should I call them our?) arms to keep them as flexible as possible. They had to put my fingers in what's called a resting hands splint because otherwise, the fingers will start curling in. And once they do, it's almost impossible to stop. My arms were splinted, too. They don't want the elbows to move. And, oh yeah, I was on about forty pills a day—immunosuppressants, magnesium, prednisone, antibacterials, antiviruses—you name it.

I stayed in the intensive care unit for three days. Then they removed the urinary catheter—*yeow*—and transferred me upstairs. (Please, don't ask me to explain that one.) And it was weird that everything was very hush-hush. There wasn't even a name on my door. Brigham, I guess, wanted to make damn sure I was okay—meaning the surgery was a success—before scheduling a press conference. It was also important to keep the date of the surgery secret—to give the donor's family the time they needed to grieve and to remain anonymous, as they had requested.

In the meantime, Jess went home and moved out of her apartment in Virginia, putting all her stuff in my house in Fredericksburg. She promised she would be back in forty-eight hours, because I had told her about the ex-wife who never returned. In fact, she drove straight from Virginia to Boston to make sure she made it and passed out with exhaustion when she finally got to the hospital. She had made the commitment to be with me full-time—hell or high water. I didn't take that lightly, and looking back, it was at that point in our relationship that the thought of marriage crossed my mind.

I should also mention that Jim and Brent were solid as well, regularly checking my mail and making sure everything was good at my house.

Just before Labor Day, I was transferred to the Spaulding Rehabilitation Hospital in Boston, not terribly far from Brigham. The folks at Brigham supplied me with a handy booklet, telling me what I couldn't eat and what I could and couldn't do. For example, I could not be around birds or reptiles or change a litter box. No worries there; as you know, I'm a dog person. They also wanted to ensure my body wouldn't reject the new arms—the biggest risk I faced, at this point in my recovery.

Well, damn, it happened anyway. No Marine preparation could have prevented it. Shortly after I began rehabilitation at Spaulding, Jess happened to notice a nasty rash developing on my arm. We called Dr. Talbot right away, and he and a nurse practitioner rushed right over. They decided to take biopsies. We didn't hear anything from them for a couple of days, then the terrible news came. "It's bad news, John," Dr. Crandell told me. "I'm afraid we have a rejection."

I totally broke down and cried my eyes out. It was like I stepped on another damn IED! I don't know why, but I thought it meant that Dr. Talbot would have to detach my new arms. That's what I thought rejection meant. But Jess called Dr. Talbot to explain my fears, and he helped her calm me down. He said it was bad, but not *that* bad. As it turned out, I had a severe grade-three rejection episode. Only a grade four is worse. Grade four can often require removal of the transplanted limbs.

So, it was back to Brigham. Dr. Talbot called in the experts—the kidney transplant doctors. They decided to treat the rejection with high doses of steroids for three days. It worked, but boy was it rough. Roid rage, I called it. My face got fat, my forehead broke out with acne, and I became really snappish. I'm sure I was no picnic to be around, but I was still rational enough to realize how supportive Jess was during all this.

Once the rejection scare passed, I could think about other things. For example, that marriage thought I had was slowly morphing into a plan for the proposal. I had a birthday coming up on September 13—the perfect time, I thought, to pop the question. After everything Jess had done for me, and how she didn't back away from some seriously disgusting things, I knew she was the one I wanted to spend the rest of my life with.

Jen, my friend I met at the Fisher House, happily agreed to help with my plan to ask Jess to marry me. She would take Jess out on a "girl's day" and steer her into a jewelry store. (Not that any woman, in my experience, would need any incentive to go to a jewelry store.) Anyway, just for fun, Jen would ask Jess to pick out a diamond ring she liked. Once that was done, the plan was to have the jeweler sneak over to Brigham with Jess's favorite rings, and I would pick one—the one I would give her for our engagement. Luckily for me, the Brigham team released me to outpatient on September 12. My plan could now be implemented and was almost fully operational.

We had already planned a trip to the Boston Aquarium for my birthday. And, luckily, they had lots of penguins there. All I had to do to execute my marriage proposal was to place Jess in front of the penguin exhibit and figure out how to present the ring to her. I was a bit worried because my fingers still weren't very functional. (Hey, I was actually playing computer games with my *nose* at this point!) Jen had also brought me four shiny rocks. Here is the symbolism: when a male emperor penguin finds the right female, he gives her the shiniest rocks he can find. If she accepts, he's got his mate!

So, I now had these rocks hidden in my hands, carefully attached with makeshift straps. The ring was hanging on the gold chain I wear on my neck to hold my cross. On cue, Jen and her daughter, Abbie, who accompanied us to the aquarium, backed away. Jess and I were standing alone in front of a bunch of those cute penguins. "Jess I have a surprise for you," I said, as I lifted my hands to show her the shiny rocks. Okay, the rock idea didn't work so great, but Jess eventually found the diamond ring. I had this great speech planned, but of course I went blank at the critical moment and forgot everything I had planned to say. Jess said, "John, you have to ask me," several times. Finally, I managed to blurt out, "Jess, will you marry me?" She said, "Yes." With the penguins as our witnesses, we became officially engaged.

We had a great time at the party we had planned later that day. Several of the folks I came to know at Brigham had set aside a suite at a hotel, so it became a great double celebration—my birthday and engagement party.

The truth was, I needed some good times, since Boston turned into a much longer stay than I anticipated, and not all of it was good. The plan had been to discharge me from Brigham as an outpatient after about three weeks. I would then stay in Boston for therapy and observation anywhere from three to six months. It turned out to be all of that—and more. Due to a series of unexpected setbacks, it would be almost February of the next year before I finally said goodbye to Boston.

Until then, when I wasn't hospitalized, Jess and I would be holed up in a long-term hotel about five minutes from Spaulding; on nice days, I could get there in my wheelchair. Thankfully, the Fisher House arranged it and paid for the first three months. It was small and had only a microwave and an electric cooktop with only two burners. But hey, we were in love. We made it work.

Boy, if only the medical part went as smoothly as our engagement. It wasn't long before I had a second rejection episode. This time, it was even worse—a more serious grade-three episode. But oddly enough, this one was easier to handle. The team again beat it with steroids.

The worst thing occurred on September 23. That night, Jess woke up in the wee hours of the morning. She felt something wet and thought it was just sweat. It wasn't. It turned out it was blood. Lots and lots of it. In fact, all of the bedsheets were soaked; we both freaked.

Jess was rushed by taxi to the Brigham Emergency Room; I couldn't go with her because the taxi wasn't handicapped accessible, but I quickly followed. They put her through a whole series of tests—about eighteen hours of them—before finally determining it was some kind of softball-sized fibroid mass. I went to the local store, bought her some coffee, a banana, and a cheese Danish. "You have been my rock throughout everything," I told her. "Now it's my turn to be yours."

Jess's surgery—a scary prospect because it could end her chances to have children—was set for November. But the time leading up to it was anything but uneventful.

First, there was that press conference on October 5 at Brigham, the one I described in the preface. I made sure there was an empty chair next to me on the dais. It's a military tradition to honor the fallen, but in this case, it honored my donor. Brigham had prepared a video of my story—from ramrod straight young Marine, to helpless quad, to new arm recipient. Dr. Talbot, with his engaging Kiwi accent, walked the audience through an animation that explained exactly how the transplant was done. Then it was my turn to speak. Even though I had been media trained, and thought I was prepared, I couldn't contain my emotions.

Fighting back tears, I said: "My deepest condolences to the family of the donor. Your loved one's death will not be for nothing. I will remember your generosity until the day I die."

Two days later, I got a curious message on Facebook. It was a photo of someone I didn't know. Here's what it said: "Hi, Sgt. Peck. Best wishes to you and your beautiful would-be wife." It was my donor's father. He and his wife had seen my story on the local CBS affiliate. They had elected to remain totally anonymous, but I guess my story moved them. They told me their son, my donor, suffered from porencephaly, a rare disease that causes cysts or cavities in the brain. He died from a cerebral hemorrhage at age twenty-seven. They said he loved cars and escalators, and at age five he played Beethoven on the piano and Aerosmith on the guitar. "Thank you for acknowledging his gift," the donor's father wrote. "He would have wanted you to have his arms." I was blown away.

I immediately wrote back to the donor's dad and asked if I could honor him on my John Peck's Journey Facebook page. He said I could, as long as I kept the family anonymous. I would honor him on November 23 and again on April 20, 2017. That would have been his twenty-eighth birthday. I would make sure I posted a message on social media, letting people know of my donor's sacrifice and what he has given to me. He literally gave me my life back. But the truth was that in my heart, I knew that I had to honor my donor every day of my life, by using his arms to help others and educating people about the importance of organ donation.

Meanwhile, I continued to learn how to use his beautiful arms. We also had time to fly to D.C. to visit friends and pick up Nasar from Jim and his family. Unfortunately, Athena wouldn't be joining us; she had failed her service dog training. She'd become too protective of her handler. And because she was no longer a service dog, she wouldn't be able to stay with us when we moved to Walter Reed after the surgery.

I was sad to see her go, but her handler stepped up and took Athena in as his own. She was in a happy home.

But my troubles weren't over. (The fun never ends when you are an amputee and a bilateral arm transplant recipient.) Later that month, a weird rash appeared on my right forearm. *Here we go again,* I thought. Dr. Talbot's nurse practitioner came over, and once again they did biopsies. This time, the diagnosis was a yeast infection. When you're on immunosuppressant drugs like I was, yeast can actually grow in places like your groin or your armpits. We treated it with a topical steroid, but the infection started to spread. Neither I nor my doctors knew it at the time, but I had poison ivy. For an arm transplant patient, that's a helluva lot scarier than just a nasty itch. And, as it turned out, it quickly got even scarier.

Jess was scheduled for surgery on November 10 at 6:00 a.m., but at 3:00 a.m. I awoke feeling really awful. I was rushed to the Brigham Emergency Room, where the doctors at first thought I might have spinal meningitis, which can kill you. Jess, of course, had to cancel her surgery. And I had to undergo a spinal tap, where they stuck a needle into the fluid around my spinal cord. Again, not something I would recommend. Fortunately, there was no meningitis. It turned out I had experienced a stress migraine, apparently brought on by my anxiety about Jess's surgery.

Finally, her surgery took place on November 22. The operation was supposed to take three hours but took more than six. The doctors removed a cantaloupe-sized tumor that weighed a whopping nine pounds. Luckily, the tumor wouldn't affect Jessica's ability to have children, which was a huge relief for both of us. The doctors would not let me return to the hotel, because with Jess laid up, there was no one to look after me. So, once again I spent the night in Brigham's Emergency Room.

Meanwhile, the poison ivy continued to do a number on me. By this time, I was beginning to suspect that was what I had, although the doctors didn't agree. I had seen plenty of poison ivy growing up in the Midwest, but it was puzzling. I had never had any reaction to poison ivy ever; hell, they even threw people into patches of it in the Marines. But whatever it was, it was definitely getting worse.

Finally, the doctors agreed with my layman's diagnosis. It turns out I was right all along! But, they wondered, how could I possibly have gotten poison ivy? The answer: from Nasar, and our walks in the park. But the weird thing was that it wasn't on my native arm. It was on the donor's. Three months after the transplant, that part of the arm—unlike my native arm —could still get poison ivy. I never had a problem with poison ivy in my entire life. And how did I know this? In the Marines, we got hazed a lot, and one of those incidences included us having to roll around in poison ivy, if you can believe that. Unlike most of my buddies, I had no reaction to it whatsoever.

So, it was really strange that my donor was so allergic. What a shocker! My donor's arms were still susceptible! It was a fascinating realization, that even though I now had two semifunctioning arms, my donor and I still had our genetic differences.

The problem with an arm transplant is that when you get something on the skin—even something as small as a bug bite—it can trigger a full-blown rejection episode, especially early on when your immune system is getting used to the new parts; that damned poison ivy triggered yet another one. The doctors treated me with the usual cocktail of high-dose steroids. They worked well at first, but then things got a lot worse.

This time it wasn't so simple, and so after hours of discussion and reviewing biopsies with Dr. Murphy and Dr. Granter in dermatopathology, Dr. Talbot and Dr. Chandraker decided to try Campath, a strong drug that basically wipes out your T-cells. A chemo nurse administered it to me intravenously.

Twenty minutes into the treatment, my heart started racing, and I had trouble breathing. I vomited over two liters of yuck. My reaction was so bad, they cut the dosage in half when they gave me the drug a week later. But the good news was that it finally stopped the rejection. Another disaster averted.

By early December, I was starting to gain control over my right elbow. And Jess and I said to hell with waiting and went to city hall to apply for a marriage license. We picked it up on December 5 and told the guy behind a bulletproof window that we wanted to come back and get married on December 9. He said there were no openings. But Jess told him December 9 was the day her grandparents and great-grandparents got married. "We wanted to honor them," she told him. I guess the guy was touched. "I'll work you two in somewhere," he told us.

So, we showed up on December 9 and waited our turn. When we were finally called, we giggled all the way through the ceremony. I'm not sure the justice of the peace was amused, but we didn't really care. After all we'd been through, we sure deserved to cut loose and have a few laughs. After we left, we celebrated our marriage with dinner at Top of the Hub, a great restaurant on the 52nd floor of the Prudential Center on Boston's Back Bay. We had beef tartare.

Jess and I celebrated our first Christmas as husband and wife in Boston. I made a sweet potato casserole in the microwave, and we cooked a Black Forest ham on the two small burners.

And on December 28—an epic day preserved on video on my Facebook page—I wiggled my fingers for the very first time! It was glorious. I wish my donor could have been there with me during that moment, but I felt his presence as I wiggled *our* fingers up and down the rest of the day. It was an awesome moment for me. Before, I was a quadruple amputee, and now, thanks to my donor, I became a double amputee. What I was sorely missing before—my ability to use my arms, hands, and fingers—was now a thing of the past. What my donor gave to me is so precious that there isn't a day that goes by that I don't think about him. That's why organ donors are heroes, in my opinion, not to mention heroes to all of the people around the world who have received organ transplants.

Speaking of Facebook, a really crazy thing happened to me right before we left Boston. Out of nowhere, I get this message from a random dude, not someone I knew personally. He told me he had no reason to live and was in the process of planning his suicide. I was freaked. Although his family had no idea what he was going to do, he told me he left for the day as usual, said goodbye to his wife and kids, went to work, and then said goodbye to his coworkers over drinks and then drove home. His plan was to kill himself later that evening. As he was leaving his home to end his life, his wife must have picked up on something in his behavior. She suggested, before he left, to check out my Facebook page because it was inspirational, and she thought that if I could have gone through all this mess, then surely her husband could find some reason to go on living. Apparently, he did, and his message to me was to thank me for giving him the strength and will to choose life instead of the grim alternative.

Wow, that was really heavy! But it goes to show how my donor's sacrifice—because of his organ donation—has not just helped me, but another total stranger, as well.

TWENTY-TWO

SERGEANT JOHN PECK, NEW AND IMPROVED

W E LEFT BOSTON AT LAST! ONLY THIS TIME, JESS AND I WERE JOINED by the arms of my organ donor, who is now as much a part of me as anyone or anything in my life. I'd like to say I was sorry to leave that place, but after all that happened in Boston, I was almost giddy at the thought of heading back to Walter Reed. That might sound strange, since being back at a military base meant I'd have to put up with some bullshit, but hey, the toughest part was behind me. And the fact remains that without Dr. Talbot and the entire Brigham and Women's team, I would have never been able to have functioning arms, let alone get my wonderful arms to do all the things I'd dreamed about. Without traveling to Boston, I might not have realized Jessica's commitment to me, or have gotten engaged and married after such a complex and difficult surgery.

The last day in Boston was uneventful. I didn't have to say any of those teary-eyed goodbyes, since I knew I would be back up there quite a bit after the surgery anyway. Jess, Nasar, and I took a cab to Logan Airport, where the three of us (four, counting my donor) boarded a flight to Reagan Airport outside of Washington, D.C. A friend had driven our van down a day earlier and parked it at Reagan. All we had to do was jam everything in and set sail for Walter Reed.

Yep, things were really looking up.

Jess and I moved into the same type of two-bedroom apartment in Building 62 that my mom and I lived in when I was there rehabilitating before Boston. We had two small bedrooms, a living room, and an even smaller kitchen in between. And to our surprise, in one of the bathrooms, we noticed a crazy sign over the toilet bowl that read: "Rainwater in Use, Not Suitable for Consumption." I guess that's a Navy thing! The apartment in Building 62 certainly wasn't spacious, but it was a big improvement over the tiny hotel room where we lived in Boston.

Technically, I wasn't even supposed to be back at Walter Reed. At the time, retired military personnel like me and their service dogs weren't allowed in Building 62 at all. But I had been working on that issue for some time. I had been going back and forth with a guy named Steve Springer, a well-connected case manager there. To this day, I don't know how he did it, but Springer pulled some serious strings—I'm talking Pentagon level—and got me and Nasar back at Building 62 to continue my therapy.

Everything was going great—at first. I was put on a regular therapy schedule, and the guys at Walter Reed were real pros. Annemarie Orr was my occupational therapist, helping me learn to use my new hands. We had met before at Walter Reed, and I liked her. She is very energetic and a caring person. Kyla—thankfully—was back as my physical therapist, working more on strengthening my shoulders and core, while keeping things lively with her usual sick humor. My other therapist, a guy—well, he was good at his job, but let's just say we didn't always see eye to eye.

I was at Walter Reed for only a couple of weeks before an organization called Wish for Our Warriors invited Jess, me, and Nasar to the Super Bowl. Can you believe it? The big game was going to be played in Houston, Texas, and, best of all, involved my favorite team—the New England Patriots. Wish for Our Warriors paid for damn near everything—airplane and game tickets, the hotel, and all our transportation. We had a great time, and luckily, my beloved Pats won in spectacular fashion over the Falcons. We also made a trip to New Orleans that February for Jess's birthday. The food was outstanding. It was important for me in my recovery to get back to doing things I did before and having some much-needed fun. While most people could never imagine how an amputee gets around, much less takes trips overseas or across the country, it's really not that bad. By this time, I was a master with my electric wheelchair. And with my new arms, it was so much easier to help Jess with getting ready for any of these excursions. I could actually pick out my own clothing, put it in the suitcase, and do all of the things I used to before with relative ease. Sometimes I would imagine how my donor used *our* arms, as well. I'm sure he did some packing of his own. But all in all, getting around now that I was only a double amputee was a breeze compared with before.

Back at Walter Reed, my therapy seemed to be progressing well, but my relationship with this male therapist wasn't. The issue this time, unfortunately, was Nasar.

One day, I think it was in March, I got a text from him. "John, don't bring Nasar to your afternoon therapy. We have a new patient who is sensitive to dogs," he said curtly in his text message. Whether that meant the dude was allergic, or the therapist just didn't want Nasar there, I don't know. But it pissed me off.

You see, there are only two things that can get a service dog kicked out of Walter Reed. The dog either isn't housebroken or doesn't respond to commands from his owner. Nasar was fine on both counts. And it turned out this therapist simply did not have the authority to ban Nasar.

Besides, Nasar was a legitimate part of my therapy. For example, in one exercise, I had to pick up a tennis ball with my new hands. I would toss it onto the floor, and Nasar would fetch. We did this over and over. But this fellow dug in his heels. He told me he would take me off the afternoon schedule if I insisted on bringing Nasar.

A couple of other things were happening, as well. By this time, there was another service dog in Building 62, and let's just say the owner was less than thorough in cleaning up after the dog. Some of the staff began blaming Nasar for the messes, even though they weren't his. It seemed like a lot of folks were looking for a reason to get rid of him. And to be fair, Nasar at this point was still an energetic, playful animal, and there were no other dogs around for him to play with. But still, he was my lifeline.

After thinking about it a lot, I made the painful decision to retire Nasar way earlier than I had planned. It really hurt me, because I loved Nasar with all my heart. But it helped a lot when my buddy, Jim Hoover, agreed to take him. Jim and his family had always loved Nasar. In fact, Nasar, the trained service dog that he is, even calmed down one of Jim's daughters when she was having an anxiety attack. His intuitive nature and love for humans made him a stellar example of what a service dog should be. Bottom line: Nasar was getting a loving family, a big yard to romp around in, and a lake to swim and frolic in. His new life would be like a summer camp all year round. It all worked out for the better, and to this day Jim sends me photos of Nasar, so I can keep up with him and still be part of his life.

It's all part of the challenges I've had to endure all of my life, especially following both of my blast injuries. I've learned—mostly through all this trauma and pain—to work through them. To take whatever life throws at you and overcome the obstacle. What other choice was there? I could succumb to the terrible life events, by simply giving up. I could become that fearful, anxious kid that the mean cop, Adam, could have created. I might go from angry kid to angry adult, thanks to my father Mike's abandonment. I could forget the Marines after my first blast. Or resign myself to life as a lonely, pitiful quadruple amputee.

I guess I'm just not wired that way. Through the incredible ups and downs of my life, there's always been that core will that survives, that never gives up no matter the obstacle, that simply will not quit. It's that tenacity and stubbornness that has helped me navigate the tumultuous life I faced. It's a curious thing. That even though I've been through hell and back, there is a part of me that is thankful for that experience. I've gone through it all and come out a better person on the other side. At least I hope I did.

The therapy, meanwhile, was generally progressing in the right direction. The therapist who had objected to Nasar decided it was best for me to work with someone else. That turned out to be Brook Walker, a very sweet and nurturing woman who helped me adapt my shower, so that I could use it by myself.

My *John Peck's Journey* Facebook page had attracted a number of followers by this time, and I tried my best to keep everyone up-to-date on my progress—especially through my homemade videos. For example, in March, I was able to show everyone how I made a Turkish-style pizza with apricot and fig chutney. I did push-ups on a yoga ball. I posted in an Iron Man Under Armour shirt. (I love dressing up like that. In Boston, I often kept warm in Deadpool and Chewbacca onesies.) There is a great benefit in comic relief of any kind when you are facing devastating injuries like mine. There are even studies that show how humor and a positive attitude can contribute to healing overall. But my bottom line for posting these videos and updates on my recovery was to show how complex our injuries are and to encourage Americans to reach out a helping hand if they are so motivated.

By the Spring of 2017, I was back in the swimming pool and attempting "real" push-ups without the ball. (I couldn't do them at that point, but

I would rip off three sets of thirty by mid-July.) In June, for our six-month wedding anniversary, I was even able to handwrite Jess the first note I ever wrote to her. It simply said: "Penguin Loves You." While the writing looked like a six-year-old's scribble, to me it was as beautiful as professional calligraphy.

Slowly but surely, I began recording many "firsts" after my transplant. The first time I fed myself with my right hand in seven years; the first time I took a shower by myself; the first time I made my own sandwich; the first time I put on my own shorts; and the first time I could do a pull-up.

There are really no words to explain what doing those simple tasks that we all take for granted—I did too before my injuries—mean to someone who is disabled. Each baby step leads to greater steps, and with persistence and determination, some functionality can and will return. What I realized at this point in my life was that before my injuries, I was just like everyone else. While I always loved helping other people, it was mostly people without visible injuries. I might have walked by a guy with no legs in a wheelchair in the past and just kept on walking. Now I'm that dude in the chair. My charitable inclinations were moving in a totally new direction.

But I wasn't just focusing on myself, my needs, and my therapy. For Christmas, Jess and I decided to contact the National Center for Children and Families. I never forgot the pain I felt as a child, when I only received a blanket for Christmas instead of a toy, drank powdered milk in my cereal, and lived in a car with my dog. So, we paid to have Boston Market cater a traditional Christmas dinner for at-risk kids, and we also made sure that they had cool presents we bought from Target under the tree.

Actually, we learned that there were two young girls and a boy who, for one reason or another, weren't on our list for gifts and would be getting nothing for Christmas. No way! Jess and I went shopping on Christmas Eve and bought the girls dolls and some nice Nike sneakers for the boy. We also had a late dinner and left our waitress a $275 tip. This last-minute stuff made our Christmas. I'd like to think that my donor would be proud of me; in fact, I know he would.

I think he also would be pleased to know just how many people on social media have been following our story. As you know by now, I didn't begin my Facebook *Journey Page* or the interviews that took place after my transplant to be famous, rich, or anything remotely like that. For me, it is always about education. One of my most important efforts has been encouraging the public to become organ donors. I even conducted an online contest where people could post their driver's licenses with their organ donation designation to illustrate how easy the process is. Because of one person—my organ donor, whose gifts were not limited to my arms—most likely six or more people's lives have been changed for the better. More dying people who are on transplant lists today would be alive if more Americans would step up to the plate.

But social media has its flip side, of course, and like everyone else, I've received some weird and negative feedback; I guess there are trolls everywhere these days. Still, the vast majority of comments have come from people I think I've touched in a positive way. They aren't always as dramatic as the guy I told you about earlier who reconsidered his plan to kill himself, but it does seem I've helped in some small way.

For that I am grateful. It's now become my life's mission.

TWENTY-THREE

PAYING IT FORWARD

HAVING MY NEW ARMS CHANGED EVERYTHING. SINCE MY BILATERAL ARM transplant, like I said, I've been able to do the simple things I couldn't do before—take a shower by myself, hold Jess's hand, and—most of all—pursue my life-long dream of becoming a chef and continuing to help others.

So, by now you know how much I love food. I was always psyched by combining ingredients to cook meals that were tasty and creative. I learned the art of molecular gastronomy, which, simply explained, is altering food as we know it, by cooking with varied temperatures and using scientific disciplines to prepare innovative meals. Things like using carbon dioxide to make foam, or liquid nitrogen to flash-freeze an item—all that fascinates me, and I'll hopefully be cooking up a storm for my family and friends someday.

But then there are the unexpected realities of life. Though my new arms are working well, there are still limitations. The most disappointing news for me was recently learning that I may never have enough strength in my arms to become a full-time professional chef. So, for the time being, I have changed course and found a new calling. Life throws curveballs at you all the time, and you have to roll with the punches, pick yourself up, and move on.

I've decided that I can do the most good by motivating others. I'm hoping to become proficient enough as a motivational speaker to be able to change people's lives by sharing my story. To make them realize that if I can get through what I have, then there is hope for them. I also want to help anyone suffering from PTSD or depression to know that there is a way out. That among all the pain and trauma they've experienced, hope can and will overcome. I'm not saying it is going to be easy, but the fact is that everyone has the power to turn their lives around. Just look at me. If I can do it, so can you.

Don't get me wrong. I still want to be a chef. I'll never stop trying, and if that day ever comes, it's off the speaking tour and into the kitchen in a flash. But until then, I'll try to be the best at whatever life brings.

So, what have I learned during this improbable journey? Well, in talking to my Marine buddies, I learned the five things to focus on: never give up; always help others; always push forward; stay positive; see the light. All of these are great, but without my relentless will, my determination to overcome everything, they are merely words. And while I'm still in my thirties, my relatively brief years, with all their challenges, have taught me some of the life lessons that I carry with me today.

There's patience, for example—a trait that was missing from my life with ADHD and the cocksure confidence of my Marine years. Along with perseverance, patience helped me push through the seemingly endless pain and trauma I've experienced since that awful day in Afghanistan.

Then there's compromise, a skill that was also totally AWOL during my Marine years. Give and take, listening to the needs of others—and giving up a little to get a lot—is the secret to living an impactful life. Jess, I truly believe, would not have liked me very much before my second injury.

I've also learned to seek my own inspiration from the right things. Like when I was first at Walter Reed planning to kill myself on the stairway. It was that wounded warrior, with his wife and child, that inspired me to scrap that plan and push through the pain. It was my donor, and my promise to his family, that inspired me to see it through.

I was always a loyal son, a dedicated U.S. Marine, and a devoted husband—and a pain in the butt sometimes, too. But when it's all said and done, the measure of any of us is what we give back to others. I've realized that simply doing random acts of kindness—though those were heartfelt—isn't enough.

Through my emerging career in public speaking, I will find ways to help other wounded warriors and all people get out of their dark spots and into something that would give them meaning, hope, and purpose. One thing you learn in the Marines is that your battle buddies come first; they are your family, in the figurative sense. Now that I have my own family—my wife, Jess, and someday a child or two—I realize that not every wounded warrior or veteran is so lucky. It pains me to know that still, twenty-two service members every day commit suicide. That isn't acceptable. One of the reasons I think this happens is that they've never left their dark spot. They come back battered—emotionally and physically—and have a tough time adjusting to civilian life. Hey, look what happened to me. I would have been one of those statistics if not for the people who were there by my side. There is always an alternative to suicide, and that is hope and having a purpose.

I am also continuing to raise awareness about the importance of organ donation; I would not be where I am today without my donor, his parents, and their sacrifice. I am continuing to publicly advocate for organ donation. It's as simple as registering your name on a variety of national websites—like the U.S. Health and Human Services (HHS) site—organdonor.gov.—or when you update your driver's license, as examples.

The HHS estimated that in 2018, there were 114,000 men, women, and children on the national transplant waiting list. In 2017, 34,770 transplants were performed, and tragically, twenty people die every day waiting for a transplant. What I found alarming is that while 95 percent of Americans support organ donation, only 54 percent actually sign up. I'm hoping to change that troubling statistic.

If not for the generosity of my donor and his parents, and the almost insurmountable odds of finding him and his arms being a perfect match, I would be a quadruple amputee for the rest of my life. And it pains me that people have to die because there aren't enough organs to help them. So, please, today, become an organ donor. Tell your friends and family, too. It's really that big a deal.

By now you know I'm no navel-gazer—meaning someone who indulges in useless or excessive self-contemplation. I'm still a Marine and pragmatist at heart. Maybe the best way to explain everything that's happened to me—and the effect it's had—is in the following analogy.

Some of the folks I've told this to don't believe me, but here it goes anyway: Imagine I found myself in a room with every damn Al-Qaeda fighter who had any part in putting that freakin' IED in my path. Now, imagine I was given permission to kill them all, with absolutely no repercussions. Would I do it?

The answer is "no." I would simply say, "thank you," and be on my way. Thank you for taking my limbs but giving me heart. That's how my bad luck has changed me for the better. It's Sergeant Peck, new and improved.

By now, you know how important paying it forward is to me. But I wouldn't have come this far if not for all of the people who taught me the life lessons that I try to live by every day. Sure, many people have had shitty childhoods filled with abuse, abandonment, and so much more. But I bet that not that many have had the added burdens of losing their memories, having all four of their limbs blown off, surviving dozens of surgeries and a rare flesh-eating fungus, two divorces, and waking up with a stranger's arms attached to theirs. Sometimes I can't even believe it myself. But from each of those challenging experiences, there were people who inspired me; what I've internalized from them is priceless. Of course, there was my mom, Uncle Toby, my battle buddies, Jess, Kyla, and many others. Though I may not necessarily connect a specific life lesson with a specific person in my life, collectively, what I have learned has helped me cope with the challenges I faced as a child, adolescent, and adult. Things like: what it means to be accountable for my actions; the importance of helping others; and to keep pushing on no matter what life throws at you. I recognized that humor can get you through the darkest days—and push through the pain—and that service is the highest calling, even if you are struggling with your own demons.

From my fellow Marines—alive and no longer with us—I realized that there is no stronger bond. From my own experience trying to find a donor and raising money for my travel to Boston, I've seen firsthand that the American people are basically generous and kind. Especially my friends and neighbors from Antioch, whose solid Midwestern values gave me the boost I needed when it mattered most. And of course, without my mom, I would never have had the strength and resilience to overcome the ravages of abuse and abandonment.

Dr. Talbot and all of the surgical team and staff at Brigham and Women's Hospital showed me people could care unconditionally, and choose to donate their time and talents to helping guys like me regain our independence.

My wife, Jess, taught me to trust again and to know that despite my limitations, I'm still a man worthy of love.

As of this writing, Jess and I have left Walter Reed, after being there for almost a year and a half. I sold my smart home in Fredericksburg because of my new lifestyle and the need to be closer to Walter Reed. We moved into an apartment to start our new life outside the confines of a medical facility.

I'm sure there will be challenges ahead—there always are—but we'll meet them head-on together.

Some of my friends have told me I've changed so much since my injuries. No kidding. I have two, new beautiful arms, a new wife, and certainly a new outlook. For the first time in many years, I appreciate the little things. A touch, a homemade meal, a warm shower and—perhaps most of all—the term *organ donor*.

So, that's my story. I hope you will benefit from what I learned and know that literally anything is possible—even for a former quadruple amputee, and someone who has had his share of abuse and abandonment, like me. I'm cool with everything. After all, those negative experiences serve to not only make us stronger but lead us to new and even better things in life. Cumulatively, all of life's experiences—both positive and negative—give us our depth and the strength to look within for happiness.

I can't wait to see how far my new attitude, Jessica's love, and my donor's arms will take me.

EPILOGUE

O N WEDNESDAY, FEBRUARY 14, 2018, I PREPARED MY FIRST VALENTINE'S Day dinner for my wife, Jessica, using our two new arms. This was my menu, courtesy of my friend and mentor and *Food Network* Chef Robert Irvine.

FIRST COURSE

ARTISANAL CHARCUTERIE AND FROMAGE BOARD
cured meats, cornichons, whole-grain mustard, country bread, assorted handcrafted cheeses, fig jam, Marcona almonds, honeycomb

SECOND COURSE

SLOW-ROASTED YELLOW BEET & BOSTON BIBB SALAD
Frisée, watercress, shaved Bosc pear, candied walnuts, champagne-Dijon vinaigrette, showered Maytag blue cheese

THIRD COURSE

ROASTED MOULARD MAGRET DUCK BREAST
French Puy lentils, butternut squash, shallots, fine herbs, parsnip puree, fermented black garlic jus

<u>DESSERT</u>

WARM SWEET POTATO BREAD PUDDING
vanilla bean ice cream, sriracha-whiskey caramel sauce

My Valentine's Day emulsion vinaigrette: three quarters cup walnut oil; one-fifth cup grapeseed oil; one-fifth cup champagne vinegar; one tablespoon honey; one minced shallot; two tablespoons Dijon mustard; salt and pepper to taste.

The main dish: one half-pound of determination; one cup of resilience; two ounces of fearlessness; three ounces of Marine spirit; and two full cups of heart.

ACKNOWLEDGMENTS

BEING A UNITED STATES MARINE IS TOUGH ENOUGH, BUT IT TAKES THE same kind of military might and precision to write a book. That is why I am grateful to so many people in my life who have helped me put my thoughts down on paper and make sense out of my unusual story. Of course, my wife, Jessica, has been a wonderful support and partner in everything. She has always been there for me and there through the dark and tough times. Jessica has been the rock when I needed it the most. With her by my side, we could accomplish anything. My mom, Norma, has supported me my entire life, and for that I am grateful. She also lent her advice and thoughts on the early parts of my life that I don't clearly remember. My thanks to my two coauthors—Dava Guerin and Terry Bivens—who have used their writing and creative talents to make this book come alive. They are true partners in this project. Mike Campbell, our wonderful editor, and the entire Skyhorse Publishing team have produced a book of which I am very proud. Dr. Simon Talbot and the staff at Brigham and Women's Hospital have been instrumental in helping me articulate the finer points of my bilateral arm transplant surgery and help readers understand the complexity and rarity of the procedure. The doctors and staff at Walter Reed National Military Medical Center have also been tremendously supportive of me and contributed to this book. Captain John Woodall (Woody) helped me recall our time together regarding the creation of the Trackchairs for wounded warriors, and so many other moments we have shared together. Woody is a hero in his own right. Gary Sinise, one of the most ardent champions of us wounded warriors, veterans, and first responders, has done more for me and others in my position than words can express. So have Judith Otter, who heads up the Gary Sinise Foundation, and Chef Robert Irvine, who has been my culinary inspiration. Frank Siller, who heads up the Tunnel to

Towers Foundation, and John Ponte have been with me all the way, and I'm thankful for their friendship and support. In fact, they partnered together with the Gary Sinise Foundation several years ago to build my first smart home in Fredericksburg, Virginia. Jennifer Griffin has always been there for me, and for that I am forever grateful. Likewise, Mary Waters from CBS News, Andrea McCarren of WUSA 9, and all of the news media who helped share my story with the world. I wouldn't be who I am today without my friends and neighbors from my hometown of Antioch, Illinois. They never forgot me or stopped supporting me. And to my battle buddies and military friends I met along my journey—you know who you are—I thank you for your friendship. And finally, to my donor and his family. Without his sacrifice and his parent's generosity, I would not be writing this book with both of my/our arms.

ABOUT THE AUTHORS

Sergeant John M. Peck

Sergeant John M. Peck (ret.) enlisted in the U.S. Marine Corps in 2005 and did two tours of duty—one in Iraq and the other in Afghanistan. In 2007, he suffered a traumatic brain injury in Iraq that left him with severe memory loss and other injuries. After overcoming those injuries, he reenlisted in 2009 and was deployed to Afghanistan. There he stepped on an Improvised Explosive Device that blew off three of his limbs and injured the fourth. He contracted a deadly fungus, and the fourth limb had to be amputated. He became one of only five quadruple amputees from the War on Terror. Undeterred, Sgt. Peck persevered through endless surgeries, and physical and occupational therapy, as well as learning to use prosthetic arms and legs. He learned about a groundbreaking bilateral and was placed on a transplant list in 2014 after a year or more researching the possibility of him being a candidate for the surgery. He was successful in that quest and in 2016 received two donor arms from a young man who died of a rare brain disease. The surgery was performed at Brigham and Women's Hospital in Boston and took two surgical teams fourteen hours to complete. Since then, Sgt. Peck has been participating in ongoing therapy and is refining his skills as a motivational speaker. He also advocates for wounded warriors. Sgt. Peck is the CEO of the John Peck Fund and a supporter of many causes, *especially* those related to single mothers and children. He resides in Bethesda, Maryland, with his wife, Jessica.

Dava Guerin

Dava Guerin is the coauthor of *Unbreakable Bonds: The Mighty Moms and Wounded Warriors of Walter Reed* (2016) and *Vets and Pets: Wounded Warriors and the Animals That Help Them Heal* (2018) both released by Skyhorse Publishing in New York. She is also the coauthor of two memoirs—*Presidents, Kings, and Convicts*, with former U.S. congressman Bob Clement (D-TN); and *Keep Chopping Wood*, with Mike Hardwick, CEO of Churchill Mortgage Corporation. She and her husband, Terry Bivens, are coauthors of *The Eagle on My Arm*, to be released by the University Press of Kentucky in Spring of 2020. Guerin is a communications consultant and freelance writer, and former communications director for the U.S. Association of Former Members of Congress in Washington, D.C. She was also president of Guerin Public Relations, Inc., a full-service communications firm, before becoming a full-time author. She was also profile editor of *Local Living* magazine and *Bucks Living* magazine; and worked in senior-level positions for Ketchum Public Relations, The Weightman Group, and the Philadelphia Convention and Visitors Bureau. She volunteers her time helping wounded warriors and their families at Walter Reed. Guerin has worked with numerous U.S. presidents and managed visits for world leaders, U.S. politicians, and entertainers. She helped launch the late former First Lady Barbara Bush's popular ABC Radio Network show *Mrs. Bush's Story Time* and supports the Barbara Bush Foundation for Family Literacy. She has also managed national and international public relations programs for many Fortune 500 companies and professional sports teams including the Philadelphia Eagles, Comcast, Tasty Baking Company; Dietz & Watson and H.J. Heinz; provided media credentialing for the 2000 Republican National Convention, the President's Summit for America's Future, We the People 200, the Congressional Medal of Honor Society, LIVE8, and the Philadelphia Liberty Medal; and was editor of the 2000 Republican National Convention's Official Delegate and Media Guide. Guerin graduated summa cum laude with an M.Ed. degree in organizational behavior from Temple University and graduated from Goddard College with a Bachelor of Arts degree in English Literature. Guerin also attended Rutgers University and the University of London's summer program focusing on history and literature. She resides in Berlin, Maryland, with her husband, Terry, and their two Labradoodles, J.P. Morgan and Tinkie.

Terry Bivens

Terry Bivens is an award-winning journalist and highly ranked Wall Street analyst. His 1991 series for the *Philadelphia Inquirer* on the Dorrance family, majority owners of Campbell Soup, was nominated for the Pulitzer Prize in 1991. His work has appeared in the *New York Times* and several business and national consumer magazines. On Wall Street, Bivens followed the packaged food industry for Bear Stearns for eleven years until the company was bought by J.P. Morgan in 2008. He was then hired as an executive director at J.P. Morgan, where he continued to cover the food industry until he retired. He is also the founder of Tasty Foods Consulting, where he counsels clients on IPOs and provides investor relations advice, as well as other financial consulting services. Bivens often appeared as a guest on television network business channels such as CNBC. He was ranked among the top three consumer analysts for many years by *Institutional Investor* and received numerous accolades for his financial work. Bivens holds an MBA from the Wharton School at the University of Pennsylvania, a master's degree in journalism from The Pennsylvania State University, and a bachelor's degree in history from the University of North Carolina. He and his wife, Dava Guerin, and their two Labradoodles live in Berlin, Maryland.